'This book has irrevocably chang[illegible]
Through succinct and often poetic [illegible]
access to glimpses of the brave, fearful, lonely and vulnerable [illegible]
of those suffering from psychiatric disorders, especially schizophrenia.
The text, illuminated by extraordinary artwork, compels one to believe
that beyond all the distress and despair, there is, and always
should be, hope.' – Antjie Krog

Madness

Stories of Uncertainty and Hope

Sean Baumann

Illustrations by Fiona Moodie

Jonathan Ball Publishers
Johannesburg, Cape Town & London

Originally published in South Africa in 2020 by
JONATHAN BALL PUBLISHERS
A division of Media24 (Pty) Ltd
PO Box 33977, Jeppestown 2043

This edition published in 2021 by
JONATHAN BALL PUBLISHERS
An imprint of Icon Books Ltd,
Omnibus Business Centre,
39-41 North Road, London N7 9DP

Email: info@iconbooks.com
For details of all international distributors, visit iconbooks.com/trade

ISBN 978-1-77619-147-5
ebook ISBN 978-1-77619-014-0

Printed and bound in Great Britain
by Clays Ltd, Elcograf S.p.A.

Contents

Introduction

This book is an attempt to make some sense of the experiences I have gained working as a psychiatrist in an admission unit of a public hospital for over twenty-five years.

Through a description of clinical encounters I have sought to address issues that I hope to be of interest but that are also problematic or contentious in the contemporary practice of clinical psychiatry. Furthermore, many of the questions that arise from these stories, I believe, extend beyond the confines of whatever might be defined as mental illness and pose concerns regarding the tenuous nature of the self, of consciousness, and of free will and community that have relevance to us all.

Another motivation has been a wish and a need to describe these encounters in a respectful and authentic way, troubled as I am by the often careless representations of madness and the harmful effects these distortions have in causing further suffering and exclusion. These misrepresentations arise to some extent from misconceptions – including, among many, that mental illnesses are untreatable or merely reflect social ills. A conflation of vaguely construed notions of self-indulgent neuroses, psychopathy and psychoses prevails among many, and in the absence of biological markers, mental illnesses are oddly considered to be not quite real.

These notions are hurtful and damaging.

A strictly biomedical approach has led to significant advances but is limited by a reductive position. Consciousness is inherently subjective, and central to any discussion of the mind and its maladies. A complementary subjective or first-person perspective therefore needs to be addressed to account for the lived experience of illness and ways of coping and finding meaning. An argument is made that meanings, however elusive, might be found in these strange stories – and, furthermore, that these meanings might be intrinsic to the process of recovery.

The categories of mental illness or psychiatric diagnoses have a limited scientific basis, and by restricting expressions of human suffering in this way we allow exclusion and limit our understanding and our capacity to be helpful.

A concern also arises in regard to the misuse of diagnoses and the inappropriate medicalisation of human suffering, thereby undermining the ability to cope with adversity. Thresholds for the diagnoses of psychiatric disorders are uncertain. Overextending the boundaries of what might be considered an illness is not helpful and can cause further harm in creating inappropriate expectations and leading to unnecessary and inappropriate treatment.

The encounters described in this book and the stories that are told to develop these themes are all authentic, and arise directly from my work as a clinical psychiatrist in the male admission service of Valkenberg Hospital in Cape Town. Names have been invented and certain details changed to respect the privacy of our patients and their families, and to respect confidentiality.

In the difficult circumstances described, I have been deeply moved and inspired and filled with hope by my engagement with our patients and their families. They demonstrate great courage and resilience in struggling with extreme and profoundly ill-understood forms of distress.

This book is an attempt to change our harmful ways of thinking about mental illness. It also seeks to pay tribute to those who live with these mysteriously altered states of mind and ways of being in our shared world.

Sean Baumann
Hangklip

Prologue

The hospital on the other side of the river

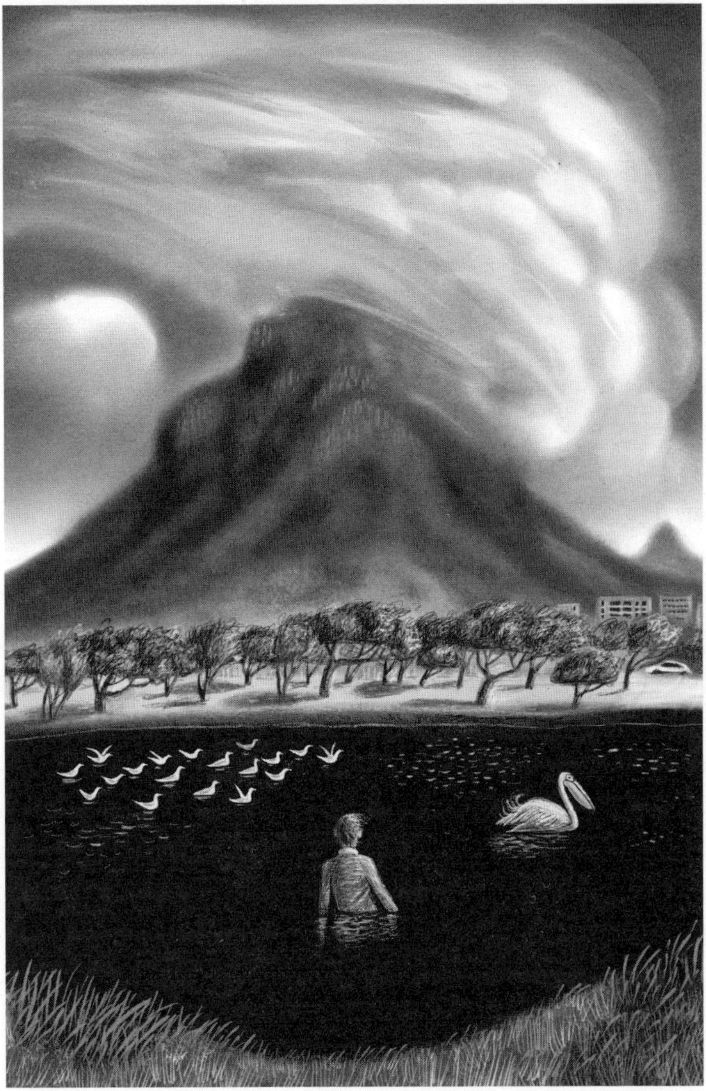

A patient is standing in the middle of the river. He is gazing across the water to the city and the mountain above where the sun is setting. His back is turned to the hospital. The nurses are waiting for him patiently on the riverbank. He seems uncertain whether to cross the river or to return. There is no danger. He is on the edge, in an in-between space, as is the hospital where I have worked as a specialist psychiatrist for over twenty-five years.

It is time to get away. The corridor is quiet. My colleagues have left. I close the laptop, as if that could shut out the clamour. I take nothing with me, hoping that this will enable me to turn my back on the events of the day. At the door of the Education Centre a voice calls out from behind the fence of the male high care unit. 'Goodbye, Doctor. Safe trip home.' The simple gesture seems to me to be an act of surprising kindness. This man has been admitted to the hospital as an involuntary patient. I am, as the treating psychiatrist, partly responsible for keeping him here. Yet he shows a generosity of spirit, not anger.

On the other, female, side of the unit, the women are ululating as if it is a party. Then silence.

The shadows of the mountain are stretching across the river and over the fence and into the grounds of the hospital. At the gate the security guard gives a cursory glance into the back of the car and smiles and waves, as if she herself is bemused by the arbitrariness of the process of crossing the threshold.

Leaving the hospital, on the right is the entrance to the observatory. Here, adjacent to the hospital, on the same side of the river and at the edge of the city, our colleagues are gazing at the edge of the universe. I imagine a great stillness, an immense calm out there, in contrast to the tumult of the hospital. I dream of a great overarching cosmic order putting into a consoling perspective the microscopic disarray of the human brain, the personal and private anguish of madness. This is illusory, I am informed; there is a swirling chaos out there that is in parallel to the frenzy of the mind in a state of extreme distress. A photograph I find in an astronomy journal of the outer edges of the universe is virtually indistinguishable from an image of the central nervous system.

The road leads away from the hospital and the observatory to a bridge across the river. The flamingos have left and so has the man standing in the river but there are flocks of gulls and ibises. The birds are motionless, their bright reflections in the evening light mirrored in the shallow water, another threshold to cross, away from the sadness and mysteries of the unit where I work.

Xolani is not responding to treatment. He is terrified, insisting that he is bewitched and that he must get away to save his life. The hospital is part of the conspiracy. Attempting to help, we are contributing to the horror of his psychosis. Rico is doing well and we would like to discharge him soon but his family say they will kill him if he comes home. They say they will hold the hospital responsible. They are exhausted and angry. Previously, on many occasions, after he is discharged he stops the treatment and he abuses drugs. His violent behaviour then becomes extreme and the family has become ostracised by the outraged and fearful community. What is to be gained by admitting him again, they demand, exasperated, if we discharge him as soon as he is well? The hospital cannot help. Nobody can help.

Nico was discharged from the unit a month ago. The parents have told me he has disappeared, they think up into the mountain. They are desperately worried and angry. He was well at the time of his discharge but they demand to know why we allowed him to leave. This has happened before but now they fear for his life. They hold the hospital responsible for his disappearance. What are we going to do now, they want to know. How are we going to find him? 'Where is he, Doctor? Tell us where Nico is!' they cry, as if I could know, as if I could undo what has happened.

There are two pastors fighting with each other on the ward. Both believe the other to be the devil incarnate. The other gods, allahs, angels and masters of the universe seem to get along with each other relatively well. Even the king of Africa and the king of Cape Town seem to have developed an amicable relationship, and it is something of a mystery as to why the pastors seem to be locked together in this hateful enmity.

Fear, rage, kindness and a curious grace ebb and flow in the confined spaces of the acute unit. We seem almost constantly to be on the edge. Mzamo insists that he does not want to die but he has no choice. The incessant voices are telling him that he must kill himself. He must do this to save his family. Our staff numbers are worryingly low, particularly at night, and despite the suicide watch the situation is dangerous. Everybody is anxious.

Moletsi simply stares at me. I cannot read him. It is something beyond fear, something profoundly indecipherable, a deeply disconcerting state of catatonia. He appears to be baffled, but that is merely what I observe – an interpretation. Another person's mental state is ultimately unknowable. That is accepted, although something that we are not inclined to dwell upon in our customary interactions with others. But this unnerves me. He is unreachable.

Last week, a pelican appeared on the river, alone. It was majestic, disproportionate, gliding in the shallow water among the smaller birds as if unsure whether it belonged on this drab stretch of a polluted river, running its sluggish course between the hospital and the squalor of the suburbs. Seemingly disdainful, it stretched its vast wings and lumbered into the sky and turned westward towards the setting sun.

It was Cassiem who was standing almost in the same place in this river some months earlier, knee-deep in the water, uncertain whether he should go forward or turn back.

A group of nurses watched him from the grass verge. It was not clear whether he intended to drown himself. He was shaking. This could be the cold, or his apprehension, but was also due to the Huntington's disease, a progressive neurodegenerative disorder that he knows will kill him.

He was staring away from the hospital, his gaze directed up towards the eastern buttress of the mountain. Everybody was waiting. There was a patient expectation that he would return to the hospital side of the riverbank. He made an enormously sad shrugging movement, as if defeated. The water is too shallow to be drowned in, and the attempted suicide was absurd and futile, a mere gesture of despair.

Perhaps he had imagined the river symbolically, and that, by immersing himself in its spiritually healing torrents, he would be carried away from the misery of his body, to the oblivion of heaven. He stood in the water, motionless, his back to the hospital, until one of the nurses cautiously entered the water and took his hand and, without a word, led him back to the verge, back to the ward, to momentary safety and a cup of tea.

Crossing the river, crossing the road, entering the suburb of Observatory, now in shadows, I find myself in fatigue, wishing and hoping that these predicaments might with distance and time begin to seem less insurmountable. This is not a particularly helpful or resourceful attitude, and, equally without reason, I imagine that in the morning I will return with a renewed vigour and hopefulness.

Observatory itself seems to be on the margins, between the hospital and the more ordered city, many of its inhabitants living precariously, just holding on, the southeasterly wind now blasting through the forlorn streets, papers dancing in frenzy, blank faces trapped in cars, people huddled in doorways, some of whom I recognise as former patients.

Rising away from the suburb, the road joins the highway and turns westward, across the shoulder of Devil's Peak towards the city. Buffeted by the increasingly furious wind, the city hovers at the edge of a churning green sea and, beyond the bay, at the edge of a vast continent.

The cloud has become a towering wave of silver in the evening light, pouring over the mountain and obscuring the ravines. The cables rising from the lower cable station disappear in the distance like frail threads into this swirling chaos. Absurdly, an image comes to me. I have taken control of the winches in the lower station. I pull the levers, release the brakes. The cables tremble and the great wheels turn. We all look upward into the churning cloud. At first, nothing. The cables strain and pull, and then gradually, emerging from the howling tumult, a figure emerges, suspended from the cable, being brought down carefully, slowly to safety. We draw him down to us. It is Nico, restored at last to his waiting family who embrace him in joyful relief. I am annoyed with myself: surely things cannot be that desperate that one resorts to this sort of wistful fantasy. And even were Nico to recover, as in all likelihood he would, it will only be a matter of time before he disappears again, lost in the mountains somewhere, back into the darkness, his parents calling in anguish, 'What have you done, Doctor? How could you let him go? Bring him back, bring back our son.'

There is a constant pressure to discharge. The male acute service where I am a consultant comprises one hundred beds. There are about eighty to one hundred admissions a month, which means we need to maintain a constant throughput, to discharge in order to admit. Earlier in the day I was informed that there were over forty people on the waiting list. These are patients who have undergone a seventy-two-hour assessment and are considered to need further hospital care, usually on the basis of a psychotic illness and some degree of dangerousness, either to themselves or to others. Usually, these patients are accommodated in units unfit for the purpose, awaiting transfer to our hospital. This causes much distress, and is a source of great anxiety and exasperation to the harried nursing and medical staff who in this casualty setting also need to attend to medical emergencies. Thus, in order to admit these very disturbed mostly young men, we are obliged to discharge patients, often before we consider them ready.

Oscar's parents want me to discharge him. He clearly remains unwell but they insist they can manage. They know him, they have been through this before, and they say that the other patients in the ward are making him fearful. I need the bed. Hurriedly I give instructions for the paperwork to be done so that he can be discharged late on the Friday afternoon. On Sunday evening he is readmitted as an emergency. Everything went well on the Friday evening and on the Saturday. On the Sunday morning, he brought his parents breakfast in bed. They thanked him and the mother asked if she could have some honey with the tea. He then pulled out a large knife from behind his back and lunged at his father. Somehow, the parents managed to wrestle the knife away from him and nobody was injured. The father later said there was some uncertainty in his movements, as if he was unsure of what he was doing.

Oscar said to us, 'I wanted to feel what it was like to kill somebody,' then later, 'I had to do it … I was following instructions.' Now he is back, and we will have to keep him for longer, but for how long?

'Doctor, we are living in fear of our lives. What is the guarantee that when you discharge him he is not going to attack us again?' Of course, there is no guarantee.

The sun has passed behind the mountain and the city is in shadow. The wind has picked up ferociously. The cloud, streaming over the mountain, disappears at the upper edges of the city and turns into an invisible torrent of wind, chasing through the empty streets and generating in many of us hurrying homeward a restless and disconcerting sense of desolation. Nothing seems substantial: all is movement and uncertainty. Everything seems precarious. After days of this relentless gale, people say, 'I can't stand it any more. The wind is making me mad.'

Stephen, whom I saw this afternoon in the outpatient clinic, has become unwell. He gazes through me, vague, perplexed. His mother phoned me yesterday to express her deep concern. He had been so well for so long that perhaps both of us, and Stephen, had begun to imagine that this was over and that his recovery would endure. He was assaulted close to his home a week ago, but even before this traumatic event his mother said that he had become increasingly withdrawn and had isolated himself in his bedroom.

'What is it, Stephen? What's happening?' A long silence ensues while he seems to be struggling to form a response. Then, making a great effort, he mumbles, 'I don't know.' He stares out of the window but he does not seem to see the birds on the river. His mind is elsewhere. There is another long pause and he mutters, almost to himself, 'No, no. Go away. It's too late. It is too late. You can't help me.'

I don't know if this is some insight on his part. I don't know whether we will be able to help him. In this profound altered state of absence recovery seems improbable. We will need to be patient. We need to have hope, but that in itself often seems elusive.

The city turns away from the hospital on the other side of the river, turning against the darkness and uncertainty and sadness as night falls, bringing with it a dream of respite, as if madness might rest.

1
The notion of madness

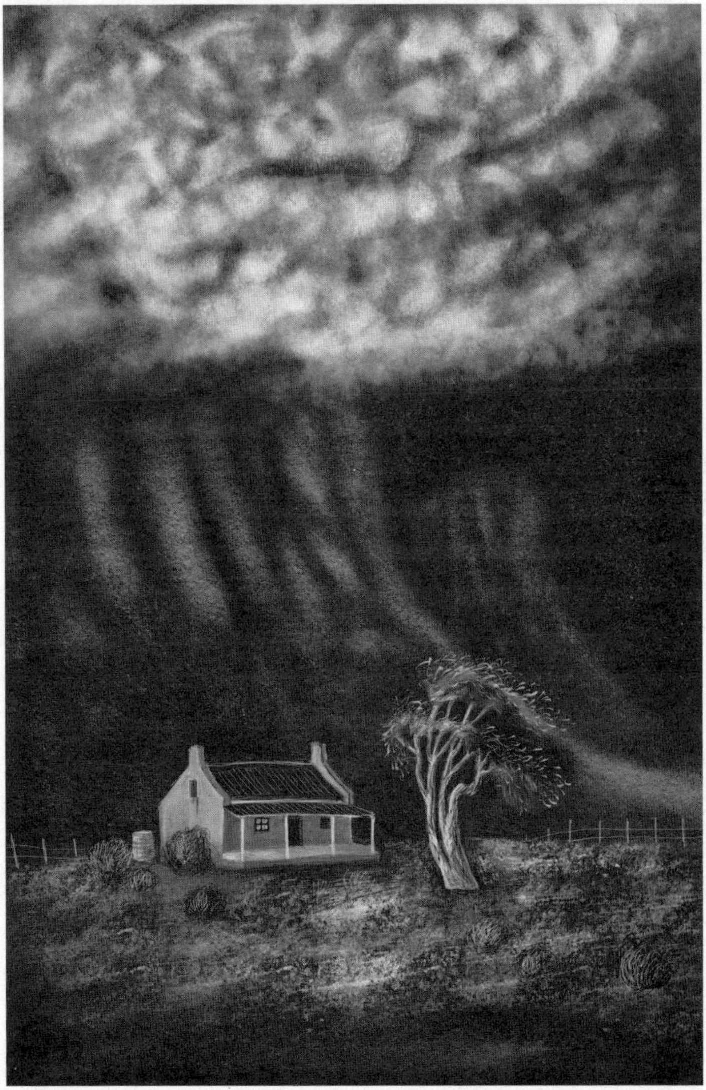

The notion of madness is problematic and controversial. Part of the problem is terminology. 'Madness' is a folk term, it is outside the conservative domain of medicine, it is fraught with metaphors. It can seem casual and flippant, and so cause hurt. The word is used here deliberately but cautiously, and with a degree of anxiety that its use might be misinterpreted as provocative.

I most certainly do not want to cause offence, and I would be dismayed if the use of the term became a source of distress to those suffering from various forms of mental illness and to their families. I have discussed this with the patients in my care. None has objected. Claude did express some concern that the term might be misinterpreted. There was in this a sense of wariness, of fatalism. It seemed to me understandable that he was sceptical, and that the use of the word 'madness' by a doctor would merely entrench its misuse, and grant an insulting and spurious authority to the dismissal and exclusion of those struggling with mental illnesses.

Perhaps it is inappropriate. Perhaps it is naïve and too ambitious, at this time, in this place. The intention is in a way to reclaim madness, to change the way we think about madness and, without being romantic or simply ignorant, to restore a degree of dignity and respect for these extreme states of mind.

If there is a problem with the term, and it is acknowledged that there is, the issue then arises as to what alternatives are available. What might be more positive, or helpful, and less negative or pejorative? 'Mentally ill' or 'severely mentally ill' in this context seems squeamish and restricts madness to the medical domain. The wish is to take the term outside the powerfully defining and confining control of medicine, to rethink madness in the hope of diminishing its otherness.

The tension or conflict in the use of the term 'madness' also applies to the terminology of mental illness. 'Mental' infers a mind–body dualism that arguably, albeit in an abstract or philosophical way, reinforces stigma and exclusion. In a prevailing materialist culture, and within the unexamined assumptions of a biomedical language, the mind is not a real thing. Things are real inasmuch as they are verifiable and tangible. The mind is intangible and therefore mysterious or ephemeral. Our fears and our joys are thus considered mere epiphenomena of the structures and functions of the brain. The search for meaning is meaningless. Loss and yearning, the love for another, the fear of death are of no consequence, mere emanations arising from fifteen hundred millilitres of a grey putty-like substance confined within our skulls.

When confronted by the complex phenomenon of chronic pain, a question that seems to arise for most doctors is whether the pain is physical or psychological. 'Physical' is real, requiring the attention and respect of the medical profession. 'Psychological' is not real, and it is therefore not clear what should be done with it. Perhaps the problem could be diverted to a psychiatrist or a psychologist. If it is psychological and not real in not having an ostensible, physical cause, where does it come from? The most obvious answer, and I don't think that this is examined critically, is that it comes from the patient, that it is made up, that it is manufactured.

The concern is not merely of terminology but of the notion of madness itself, and a large part of this – and the burden of this – is the otherness of madness. To say something is mad is to dismiss it. To say somebody is mad is to suggest a difference of a fundamental nature, deserving or requiring exclusion. Madness defines our reasonableness, our sanity. It reassures us of our normality. Inclusion requires exclusion, needs fences; boundaries need to be defined to keep at bay the roaming threats of unease and uncertainty. The notion of madness is a useful strategy for compartmentalising and displacing these difficult parts of ourselves, these unfortunate concomitants of human consciousness. In these respects, madness is a vague, amorphous concept, a necessary, virtually inevitable abstraction.

At a more pragmatic level, and veering more towards the less emotionally charged language of medicine and psychiatry, the term 'psychosis' is often used. This itself is open to debate, and defined in various ways. It might indicate severity, suggesting a continuum or a spectrum ranging from a mild disruption of the soothing tide of events to the calamity of psychosis, or madness. It might also indicate specific phenomena, most characteristically delusions and hallucinations. Of concern, and particularly with regard to the notion of otherness, is the extent to which these phenomena are considered qualitatively different. Is madness a matter of degree, a merely quantitative issue, or is it a more fundamentally, qualitatively different affliction? Conceptualising madness as a matter of degree, on a continuum with what we would regard as consolingly normal, would surely undermine – if not dispel – the notion of the other, the terror of madness and its deplorable consequences.

This is not merely rhetorical. It is a question that can be answered by considering the evidence. This evidence shows that a significant proportion of young people in particular, during the period when schizophrenia is most likely to manifest for the first time, describe psychotic symptoms in the absence of any sign of illness. Symptoms therefore need to be delinked from syndromes, but this does not happen. Hearing voices or being deluded is perceived as equalling psychosis, or madness. A young person, perhaps in stressful circumstances, complains of hearing a voice when nobody else is present. An assumption of psychosis is made, or of a severe mental illness, and the person becomes a patient. This can be the beginning of a long, fraught and contested process – long because mental illnesses are considered chronic disorders, fraught because the young person has become identified as being ill, and contested because, of course, this identity is rejected. In the turbulent environment of an outpatient clinic, and more probably in the public sector, the necessary caution and patience are rarely exercised. Simply being watchful is not considered an option, or is deemed negligent, as in recent years a persuasive argument has been made for early intervention, with the claim that the duration of an untreated psychosis is associated with poorer outcomes.

Another fairly similar argument for regarding psychotic symptoms on a continuum, and not necessarily as inevitably or intrinsically indicative of pathology, is the recognition that we all, in certain circumstances, have the capacity to experience psychotic symptoms. Sensory deprivation, certain illnesses – particularly febrile states and metabolic disorders – and a wide range of medications and psychoactive substances can trigger psychotic symptoms. Surely many of us have had the painful experience in bereavement of hearing the voice or feeling the presence of somebody who is no longer with us.

It might be useful to interpret these curious phenomena in the light of current neuroscientific thinking in an attempt to diminish the otherness, the stigmatising pathology, of these altered states. Light is without colour. The redness of the apple is not inherent in the apple. The colour of red is generated in my mind as an outcome of a series of complex processes beginning with light waves of various frequencies, but without colour, impinging on the rods and cones of my retina. This same apple is without taste or flavour until it enters my mouth and its pungency activates taste buds and olfactory cells. These sensory experiences are complex and intensely subjective. The redness of the apple I perceive is not the redness you perceive. To some extent we all live in our own worlds. To some extent we all make up our own worlds, anyway. That is not madness. Either we need to come to terms with a possibility that we are all in some ways a little bit mad, which is a cliché, or we need to consider a much more inclusive, less discriminating attitude towards experiences we do not share or understand.

In the early part of the eighteenth century, the Irish priest and philosopher George Berkeley posed the enigmatic question: if a tree falls in the forest and nobody is there to hear it, does it make a sound? Three hundred years later, there seems to be a degree of convergence between philosophers and neuroscientists as the answer to this question, which is no. There is no sound because it is not perceived. Perceiving brings the world into being; it appears that this is a general principle, one not confined to the mad.

William was brought to the unit in an agitated state. He was accompanied by the police, to whom he had fled in terror. He was from upcountry and had come to the city in the hope of finding inspiration. He was an artist, a poet, and had been struggling to develop a creative focus. He had found the city distracting, so he had rented an isolated cottage on the coast, about an hour away from the hospital. There, on his own, he sought – in a state of increasing anxiety – to retrieve the creativity that he told us gave meaning to his life.

Towards evening, the wind had risen. I am familiar with the area. The wind comes roaring and howling down the mountain in fitful bursts of a quite extraordinary force and intensity. In the growing darkness, against the slope of the mountain, this wind created in the cottage intermittent moaning, keening sounds that, as night fell, filled William with an increasing sense of dread. It was a sound that was completely unfamiliar to him. It could not possibly be simply the wind. Something else was happening, something much more sinister and foreboding.

There was no electricity in the cottage and the only illumination was created by a flickering candle. In this subdued light, he perceived what he initially thought were shifting shadows on the wall. Becoming increasingly fearful and disoriented by the wind and the darkness, he formed a ghastly apprehension that these shapes were not shadows but stains, and that the stains were of blood. He realised with horror, then, that the mournful sounds that had been tormenting him were not the wind but the pitiful cries of infants in great distress. These laments seemed to emanate from above him, in the loft area below the roof of the cottage. His senses increasingly deranged, but in a desperate attempt to trace the source of his distress, he found a ladder and climbed into the loft. Here, in virtual darkness, he gazed in horror on a mass of bleeding, mutilated children, some dead, some crying out to him, their blood copiously flowing and seeping down the walls of the godforsaken cottage. He fled, somehow found his car in the darkness and raced to the police where he gave a frenzied and incoherent account of what he had encountered.

It was almost immediately assumed that he had lost his mind, so he was brought in the middle of the night to the hospital. When seen by the doctor on duty, it was apparent that his great distress was intensified by the realisation that the police were not going to act on the information that he had given them and rescue the children. To add to his horror, he understood that they thought he was mad.

Later, in conversation with William, it was evident that he was an extremely intelligent and imaginative man who used his talents creatively in the composition of poetry. A number of issues had started to trouble him, including conflict with a girlfriend and financial difficulties. He sought to escape, to clear his mind, he said. On that terrible night, he acknowledged that he was not himself. He could not make sense of the bewildering sounds yet, partly because of his vivid imagination, he felt compelled to investigate. Not knowing what was happening, in the storm of the outside world or within himself, was a cause of anguish. He had to have an answer, however dreadful it might be.

There was another memorable encounter with William after he had recovered. I was involved in making a documentary about schizophrenia and I asked him whether he was prepared to talk on camera about what had happened to him. He agreed enthusiastically. He wanted us to know what it was like. We took him to a sound studio. The engineer created a range of sounds for him to identify which ones most closely matched the quality of his hallucinations. I have an abiding memory of him dancing about the studio, delighted that the particular sound had been created – and that we now knew what he had experienced, that he was no longer isolated by it, that it was shared.

It had been a madness, but it was also in some way understandable. Part of the problem contributing to the burden of stigma is the notion of madness or psychosis being intrinsically un-understandable, and therefore beyond or outside us and fundamentally other. The question must arise as to whether this is inevitable, that it is part of human nature and that the need for the other in a way represents our own failure of imagination.

This tension between a continuum or a spectrum and a dichotomy or polarity is not, of course, limited to mental illness. In the fields of sexual politics there has been a fairly recent shift away from a binary construct of male and female genders, with an understanding of the distress experienced by those who do not fit into these simplistic and inadequate categories. This pertains also to race and class, and any other way in which we might identify ourselves or become confined.

It is not clear why this does not extend into the domain of madness, and whether or not there is an equivalence, or whether some other, unknown force drives the apparent need to construct madness, with all its avoidable and lamentable consequences.

2

The need for the other

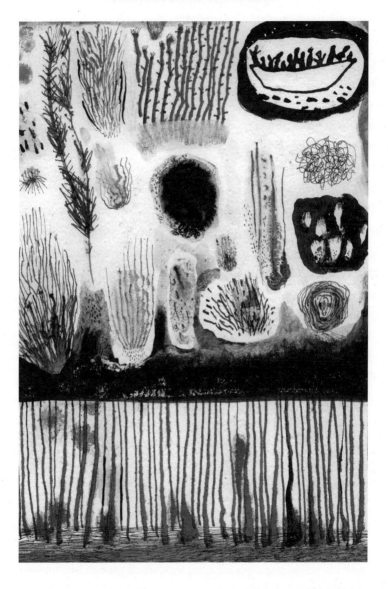

Despite a wide range of determined efforts to counter it the problem of stigma persists. 'Psychoeducation', of both the family and the 'client', are considered mandatory in the management of schizophrenia. Students and specialists in training are taught this. Research is presented to dispel the notion that madness is associated with violence. Evidence is shown that a large part of the suffering of those living with schizophrenia is due to stigma, or the exclusion that arises from this.

This phenomenon prevails, possibly to a varying extent across cultural and socioeconomic class divisions, perhaps with varying degrees of intensity, and with different consequences. It is difficult to account for this tenacious problem. It does not seem to be a matter simply of information: there seems to be a need for the other.

Valkenberg Hospital continues to appear in the imagination of many in the city as a place of fear and dread. '*Jy is mal: jy hoort in Valkenberg*' (You are mad: you belong in Valkenberg) persists as a refrain of dismissal and alienation. You don't count. You are not one of us. You don't belong with us. You are too different. You threaten us. You need to be put away – anywhere, but away from us, beyond the gates of the city, across the river.

Being away, outside, appears to be the priority. What might happen within these zones of exclusion is of lesser consideration. The driving concern is not care but separation, as if madness is contagious or contaminating. This has a particularly harsh and tragic resonance in South Africa. Many factors contributed to the emergence and persistence of the apartheid system, but a central driving force seems to have been fear: particularly, fear of the unknown, of contamination by the heathen, and of loss of land and privileges and, with regard to madness, the loss of the fragile faculty of reason.

The asylum was not created simply out of fear. A genuine concern for the mentally ill cannot be dismissed as a motivating concern, but the physical exclusion that this entailed was, in all probability, a powerful perpetuating factor. Causes and consequences become confused. It would be simplistic to argue that the problem of stigma is a consequence of the exclusion represented by the development of the asylums in Europe in the eighteenth century. The more recent trend towards de-institutionalisation, again motivated by a complicated range of factors and not solely by a benevolent concern for the mentally ill, has not, I believe, significantly reduced the burden of stigma.

Some of the difficulties in making sense of the notion of the other might be a consequence of this being regarded as an entity rather than a complex phenomenon arising from a range of interacting sociopolitical, cultural, historical and, importantly, psychological factors. We need to consider the construct in this multidimensional way if anything is to be gained in reducing its apparent intractability.

The notion of the other confers an illusion of safety, of order, of normality. There is a paradox in the need to invoke a threat in order to feel secure. Otherwise, what is there? Is all contingent, wide open, endlessly vacant, with no fence to demarcate the boundaries, to define who we might be? In early Cape Town, the wild almond hedge was an entangled, haphazard, physical expression of an edge between an enlightened European settlement and a savage darkness. The Liesbeek River is an edge between the ordered, managed and manageable city, and disorder, the imagined turmoil and the threat of madness.

We take something away from ourselves – excise something deemed inconsistent with a notion we have of ourselves – and put this something elsewhere, on the other side of the fence, of the river. We should then be safe. But the early settlers described the unease of gazing from a precarious fortress upon the campfires of the local herders they gradually began to perceive as hostile. The campfires encroached, became menacing. Lines were drawn. The fortress needs an enemy, an assailant, to justify its being. The wild almond hedge was hopelessly inadequate.

The journals of Jan van Riebeeck describe an ambivalent, uncertain, shifting attitude towards the local inhabitants. The relationships are at times cordial – cooperative, if not wary – and at other times hostile. Over the years there is a drift towards enmity, growing on one side due partly to the theft of cattle and, on the other, the dispossession of grazing lands. There were quite possibly some moments of peace, some notion of coexistence, of mutual benefit and a shared future. At what point – though surely there was no point, so over which period of time – did this possibility fade? When and how, quite imperceptibly, does the enemy become the enemy, does someone become the other?

The city gazes across the river towards the hospital with some ambivalence, if not unease.

Why the fences? Is this for the protection of those within or without? The boundaries are porous and arbitrary. Our patients wander into the suburb of Observatory and they wander back. The average length of admissions is three to four weeks. Patients are discharged; often, after a while, they come back. Families, students, workers and staff come and go. The hospital is not a fortress. Yet the divide persists, and it seems possible that in part this might be because it is intangible.

The fort, the fence, the river, all appear to be frail barriers against the unknown. A fence surrounds the hospital on one side of the river. On the other side of the river, fences, high walls, barbed wire, alarms seek to protect the houses of the suburbs. The enemy is not on the other side of the river; he or she is roaming the streets of the suburbs. The fences are not working. There is no safety. The enemy is free to roam.

At the time of writing, the city is preoccupied with a court case that involves a horrifying and bewildering family murder. It bears a disconcerting resemblance to a fairly recent murder case that gained international attention. The current case is unresolved, but the accused is a family member. In the earlier event, the accused was the partner of the lover he was found guilty of murdering. Both cases involved extreme violence – in one, the use of an axe; in the other, a shotgun. Repeated blows, repeated shots, as if the sheer frenzy and brutality of the murders signified something beyond the killing, as if the murders were an endpoint of what was described as a mounting rage and, of course, a madness.

The two murders bear a resemblance in another troubling respect. The attacks were claimed to have come from the outside. In the one circumstance, the convicted murderer claimed that he had acted on the conviction that the person he had shot was a potential assailant who had entered the apartment. In this belief, he said, sobbing, he had killed his lover. In the other, the suspected killer claimed that it was not him: an intruder had murdered his family with an axe. A middle-class family, it is claimed, is destroyed behind the high walls in the illusory safety of their suburban home by an invader. A cruel detail is added, to enhance the thrill of horror: the man is laughing as he hacks the family to death. This is an ancient story, a terror haunting the imagination for over three hundred years. The barbarians have broken down the fence and are swarming over the walls. The defences are overwhelmed. There is a terrifying sense of inevitability about the attack. Now it is upon the cowering lover hiding behind the bathroom door, the innocent, bewildered family in the safe house in the secure estate. But the attack is not from the outside, it is from within, and this poisons our consciousness with a deeper, more insidious fear. The threat from within is intolerable. Let it come from outside, if it must. The danger beyond the fence, on the other side of the river, outside the fortress, is at least more understandable, knowable. From within, like a madness, emanates another kind of fear.

Currently, Western Europe is preoccupied with the issue of immigration. This is a major item in national elections and dominates current affairs. It is a cause of intense debate. Anxious reference is made to a 'way of life', 'national identity' and 'terror'. Sometimes made explicit, more often not, is the notion of a threat, of an engulfing wave. This threat is perceived as unstoppable. No international law, no policeman on the shore, can stop the tide. The fear is spread wide. Now it comes not across the fence, the river, but across the ocean, in broken, leaking boats. The fear provokes reaction. There is a rise in extremist, nationalist politics. The barricades go up. Invocation of the other, a threat to a way of life streaming across borders, has become a useful tool for gaining political support.

A wide range of factors contributed to the formation and the maintenance of the apartheid system for most of my childhood. The monopoly of power and wealth in disregard of justice were powerful perpetuating factors, as was, perhaps less obviously, fear. A fear that, persisting over the centuries, unabated, gathering force and hammering at the gates of the apartheid edifice, developed a relentless momentum. Confused with this fear was an ambivalence, an uncertainty, as to who or what constituted the other. A mutual dependency confounded customary notions of difference. Exclusion was ineffective. White babies clung to the backs of their black carers. All over the country, townships were situated away from the city, but not too far away. Smoke from the wood-burning fires of the workers' corrugated-iron dwellings would have been visible from the town on the other side of the hill or koppie, exciting ancient fears.

These contemporary but desperately poor settlements were separate, but not too separate to be out of mind. A dependable supply of labour was needed. Racial segregation became inefficient, impractical and impossible, yet continued to hold sway as a hollow or cynical political slogan. The other was necessary, politically expedient – but now, the other became gradually less other and lost definition. What to do? Would it be imaginable to be without the need for the other? How necessary, after all these years of an accustomed way of thinking, a habit of fear, is the other in order to define us?

Mtembe is admitted to the unit in a floridly psychotic state. The family seem curiously unperturbed. He has been bewitched. It is clear. He has had some success in a business venture and this has provoked the envy of others. Arrangements have been made. Money has been spent and the evil spell cast. Our task is simply to make Mtembe better. The use of standard antipsychotic medication to achieve this does not trouble the family. We are not required to provide an explanation; the explanation is consistent with cultural beliefs. Any talk of a biological contribution and certainly a genetic disposition is meaningless and alien. His madness does not pose any threat. The attribution to witchcraft resolves that potential difficulty. Witchcraft as a way of making sense of something that might have caused terror is therapeutic, if not for Mtembe then clearly for his community. The other has been named, and so loses its dreaded force. The serpent loses its fangs. Mtembe is not excluded because he appears to be mad. The provision of a culturally meaningful explanation renders the invocation of the other unnecessary.

Perhaps those on the other side of the river are not dangerous. Perhaps, with some bartering, some friendly cooperation, some sort of dialogue, difficulties might be resolved. Differences might not be insurmountable. Perhaps the enemy is not the enemy.

An attempt to explain the persistence of stigma, the apparent need of the other through recourse to historical events, might seem extravagant or absurd. It might be argued that the notion of the other is simply part of human nature, but what is possibly more mysterious is the persistence of the need for the other. It has been suggested that stigma arises to some extent from fear, and that this fear concerns the apprehension of the other that becomes all the more menacing as it is unknown and unfathomable. Defining the other, labelling it in whichever way might be convenient and meaningful to both the patient and the community, at least mitigates the unease. It is also probable that the stigma attached to mental illness has less to do with the nature of mental illness, or madness, itself than with the perplexing need for the other.

Why the other should be a source of fear and apprehension anyway is in itself curious. God is unknown and worshipped. The ineffable, the transcendent, the hidden order of things are endowed with a positive, enhancing spiritual quality that has been a source of yearning throughout history. Is it impossible that madness, rather than being a source of fear and hence exclusion, could require the need or wish to learn, to understand, to extend our notion of who and how we might be in the world?

This is less an issue of knowledge than of the need for a fundamental change in attitude. We cannot assume that acquiring knowledge in some automatic way changes attitudes or enlightens. How do we allow it in ourselves to perpetuate the burden of stigma? Are our notions of our own sanity so tenuous, our beliefs in the order of our world so precarious, that we regard the need for the other as inevitable?

3

The frontier: A historical context

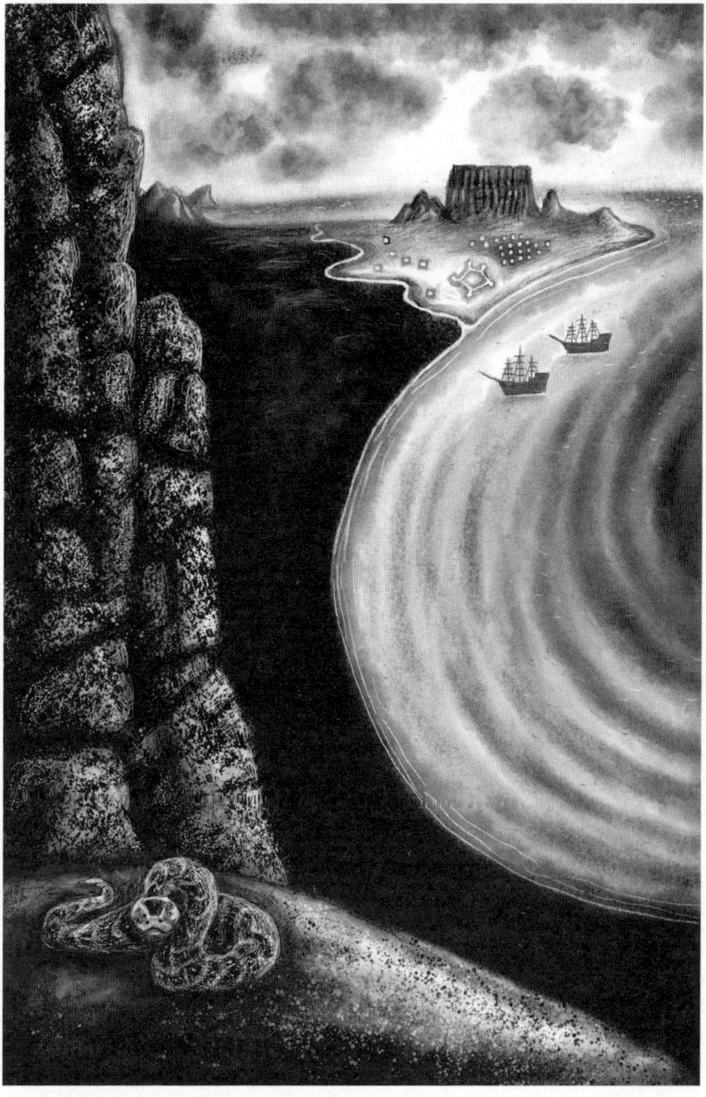

The Liesbeek River arises on the eastern slopes of Table Mountain above Kirstenbosch National Botanical Garden. It flows through the suburbs of Bishopscourt and Rondebosch to Observatory, where it joins the Black River, and ends in Paarden Eiland, absorbed into the Atlantic Ocean of Table Bay. This is the Cape of Storms, or the Cape of Good Hope. It is in Observatory that the river drifts past the hospital, dividing the hospital from the city.

It is not a long river, its course being approximately nine kilometres. It is for the most part shallow and clogged with the reeds that give it its name. It is not grand. It is an improbable frontier, this thin, inauspicious stretch of water that marks the start of the colonial project in southern Africa, that heralds the dispossession and the conflict that have endured from the middle of the seventeenth century to the present day.

If dispossession is central to the way in which the conflict is understood, the year 1657 might be considered as the beginning of this long history of strife. In October of that year, Jan van Riebeeck – directed by the VOC (the Vereenigde Oostindische Compagnie, or the United Dutch East India Company) governors in the Netherlands – granted freehold lands along the Liesbeek to a number of the company's employees. This was motivated in part by the need to control costs in the savings gained by not paying wages, but also by the need for fresh food for the garrison and the passing ships in Table Bay, and in the belief that this might be more efficiently produced by private enterprise.

A number of violent confrontations between indigenous groups and European adventurers had preceded this date. In 1510, following what seemed to have been a botched kidnapping, Francisco de Almeida, the first viceroy of the Portuguese Indies, was murdered with fifty of his men by the Khoikhoi. De Almeida had ostensibly approached the Khoikhoi pastoralists somewhere in the Liesbeek valley to barter for sheep and cattle. It is not clear what ensued or why the Portuguese attempted to kidnap the two Khoikhoi. There was an altercation. It escalated. The Europeans were violently assaulted, and apparently in seeking revenge were murdered. It is not clear whether an initially potentially cooperative encounter could have been resolved peacefully, or whether this violent outcome reflects an inevitability in the clash of European settlers and agriculturists and local pastoralists, a conflict that, in its various permutations, persists to the present. Nor is it clear to what degree arrogance, fear, greed and stupidity – and, in the prevailing thinking of the times, a careless dogma of divinely ordained superiority – contributed to this harbinger of turmoil.

Thereafter, the local inhabitants were portrayed by the Europeans as barbarians, as dangerous and heathen savages, the embodiment of the terrifying other.

> Of all people they are the most bestial … they are the reverse of human kind … so that if there is any medium between a rational animal and a beast, the Hottentot lays the fairest claim to that species … they are as squalid in their bodies as they are mean and degenerate in their understandings … their native inclinations to idleness and a careless life, will scarcely admit to either force or rewards … their common answer to all motives of this kind, is that the fields and woods afford plenty of necessaries for their support, and nature has amply provided for their subsistence … so there is no need for work … and thus many of them idly spend the years of a useless restive life.[1]

This contempt conflicted with need. The Dutch were sick and starving, gazing with hope and envy and fear upon the herds of the Khoikhoi, moving into the fertile valley of the Liesbeek for pasture as part of a tran-

1. John Ovington, master of the *East Indiaman Benjamin*, quoted in Raven-Hart, R. (1970). *Cape of Good Hope 1652 to 1702: The First Fifty Years of Dutch Colonization as Seen by Callers*. Cape Town: A.A. Balkema, cited in Mostert, N. (1992). *Frontiers: The Epic of South Africa's Creation and the Tragedy of the Xhosa People*. London: Jonathan Cape, p. 107.

sient nomadic rhythm. Hope would have arisen from an expectation that they would be able to barter for sheep and cattle, the wealth of these 'bestial vermin', and fear from the notion of the other, the encroaching hordes on the banks of the river, the campfires at night, and what must have seemed the vulnerability of the fort on the edge of an unknown continent. Fear, then, existed on both sides of the river: on the west side, of death by starvation or violent attack, of annihilation and also, perhaps, the anxiety of being alien, of being too far away, of dislocation; and on the east side, on the side of a vast continent, the dread of dispossession, of the beginning of an end.

Stigma is a complex phenomenon, and a wide range of factors contribute to its mystifying endurance, given the amount of information available to support its damaging effects. It would, of course, be simplistic and inappropriate to consider the events described here as in some way causative, but it can be argued that ignorance – and, arising from ignorance, distrust and thence exclusion – are significant historical and cultural factors that shape the local expression of this iniquity that contributes greatly to the suffering of those deemed mentally ill.

An instance of this ignorance and its calamitous consequences emerges from the beginnings of this engagement on either side of the river. Van Riebeeck is confounded. His men are quite desperate. They see the ample herds of sheep and cattle across the river and cannot understand why the pastoralists are unwilling to barter.

In frustration and with disdain, Van Riebeeck records in his journal: 'Would it matter so much if one deprived them of some six or eight thousand cattle? For this there would be ample opportunity, as we have observed they are not very strong.'[2] Almost from the beginning of the arrival

2. Thom, H.B. (ed.). (1952). *Journal of Jan van Riebeeck, Volume I, 1651–1662.* Cape Town: A.A. Balkema, p. 16.

of the Europeans on the southern edge of the continent, a delineation of power on either side of this slack, inconsequential river is established, the notion of harmonious coexistence is set aside, and the resort to force is proposed as a solution – as if this is reasonable and just. For the time being, Van Riebeeck is constrained by the company, and urged to barter rather than seek war.

There is, from the start, a failure to understand that, for the Khoikhoi, livestock – not land – represents wealth. There is a further and dangerous misapprehension regarding the occupation of land in the failure to recognise that the land occupied by the company employees forms an integral part of the pasturage routes of the Goringhaiqua and the Gorachoqua. The marine shoreline also provides subsistence for the Goringhaicona, and the Cochoqua move their grazing routes south from the Swartland during the summer grazing pastures in the Liesbeek valley.[3] The VOC settlements lie in the path of these routes. The Khoikhoi pastoralists cannot fathom why a vastly wealthy company, recently arrived from a distant country, should assume any right to impede their movement, and the settlers – with a different notion of land ownership, combined with a belief of racial superiority – are affronted by the failure of the Khoikhoi to acquiesce. They are also in all likelihood in fear of their lives.

In 1657, with these increasing pressures on land and with tensions rising, Van Riebeeck persuades the VOC to allow a number of its servants to be released from the company and establish themselves along the banks of the Liesbeek as free burghers. This is the moment at which Cape Town becomes a settlement, and is no longer a mere refreshment station. The lands on the west side of the river are occupied, owned. A frontier is established; an edge is defined.

---

3. Worden, N., Van Heyningen, E. & Bickford-Smith, V. (1998). *Cape Town: The Making of a City*. Cape Town: David Philip.

The Khoikhoi pastoralists demand to know where they are to graze their cattle. Van Riebeeck suggests that they move inland, to the north and west, but this puts them at risk of conflict with the Cochoqua or Saldanhars and the proposal is rejected. A leader of the Goringhaiqua or Kaapmans, Chief Autshumato, is lured to the fort on the shores of Table Bay and a hundred of his cattle are captured by the Dutch. One Kaapmans is shot dead and another wounded. Autshumato is dispatched to Robben Island, from where he escapes eighteen months later. The Kaapmans respond by stealing the free burghers' cattle and burning their homesteads. The two sides are effectively at war.

On 19 May 1659, the council of which Van Riebeeck is head meets at the fort and issues a declaration that will set the country on a path of conflict and acrimony and mistrust for the centuries that are to follow:

> Since we see no other means of securing peace and tranquillity with these Cape people, we shall take the first opportunity practicable to attack them with a large force, and if possible, take them by surprise … we shall capture as many cattle and men as we can … the prisoners we shall keep as hostages, so that we may restrain and bring to submission those who may evade us … the council prays that it may please the Lord God to attend us with His Blessing and His Help. Amen.[4]

In his journal, Van Riebeeck reports on and dismisses the grievances of the Khoikhoi:

> They strongly insisted that we had been appropriating more and more of their land, which had been theirs all these centuries, and

4. Resolution of the Council of Policy of the Cape of Good Hope, 19 May 1659, C. 1, pp. 423–428. Available at http://databases.tanap.net/cgh/.

> on which they had been accustomed to let their cattle graze. They asked if they would be allowed to do such a thing supposing they went to Holland … and 'as for your claim that the land is not big enough for us both, who should in justice rather give way, the rightful owner or the foreign intruder?' Eventually they had to be told … that their land had fallen to us in a defensive war, won by the sword, as it were, and we intended to keep it.[5]

This was the justification of dispossession and ruin by force. There is no attempt to provide a moral argument. Perhaps there is no sense of a need; God was considered to be on the side of the Europeans, as it was assumed that there was divine support for the fateful election of the Nationalist government almost three hundred years later. So there was no further need to accommodate, no need for compromise, no need for sharing, no more need for caution: to the victor went the spoils of war.

The other having been defined and conquered, exclusion of course had to be established and maintained and defended. A series of palisades and watchtowers were erected along the banks of the river, with a system of flag-signalling to the fort to warn of danger. In addition, the planting was ordered of a wild almond hedge and other fast-growing brambles and thornbushes to prevent intrusion and to protect the settlers' land and cattle. These were the precursors of the high walls and the barbed wire that have become a feature of present-day, predominantly white South African suburbs.

Flags, bitter almonds, barbed wire: it seems impossible to imagine that these frail measures would provide an adequate degree of security or peace of mind, as if the exclusion of the mentally ill could bring the fear of madness under control, as if being safe and normal were possible. Yet

---

5. Thom, H.B. (ed.). (1952). *Journal of Jan van Riebeeck, Volume I, 1651–1662*. Cape Town: A.A. Balkema, pp. 195–196.

at the time of writing, and for the foreseeable future, the sluggish Liesbeek River will divide the hospital from the city, and in this division perpetuate the fear of the unknown and the stigma of mental illness.

The unknown does not necessarily generate fear. Wonder at the unknown seems entirely possible, and may be one way of coping with the uncertainties of life and the mysteries of the universe. If Valkenberg Hospital represents an edge of sanity and order, and a space for the examination and treatment of the turbulent inner workings of the mind and brain, another adjacent institution, separated from the hospital by a narrow gravel path, turns outwards to examine the edges of time and space.

The first permanent observatory was developed on the site adjacent to the hospital in October 1820. From this point on the edge of the river – at the time menaced by venomous snakes (the rocky mound on which the observatory was erected was initially named Slangkop) and surrounded by leopards and hippopotami – the shape and edge of the southern hemisphere were determined and the mass of the moon and Jupiter were measured. The distance of the sun from the earth was estimated, and this remained the standard for nearly half a century. In the later part of the nineteenth century the observatory was involved in a major international effort to produce a detailed photographic 'map of the heavens'.

Order, precise measurement and, in this scientific ambition, the control of chaos is brought to the edge of the river and the city and the continent. On either side of this narrow gravel path, but on the same side of the slow drift of the river, two city institutions coexist – one turned inwards to the turmoil of the mind, seeking illumination to aid recovery, and the other turned outwards, searching through measurement to find order in the chaos of the universe.

Visitors to the city are surprised at twelve o'clock each day (with the exception of Sundays) by a loud explosive retort that reverberates across the city bowl, a booming echo of assault. In a flash and a puff of smoke there occurs momentarily a memory of danger. The pigeons in the Company's Garden rise from the oak trees in an agitated flock, having no such memory. There seems to be nothing to confirm this, no sustained clamour of violence, and the birds return to the trees and the city resumes its customary rhythms.

This reed-clogged river, emerging from the southern slopes of Table Mountain and flowing slowly through the southern suburbs of the city, past the hospital and the observatory to join the Black River and enter the sea in Table Bay, is a centuries-old frontier. It represents a margin, historically, of a European settlement, of a claim of ownership and dispossession, and the beginning of enduring conflict and mistrust. It persists as an edge, on one side of the gravel path, of measuring time and space – and, on the other, of the precarious notions of sanity and madness.

4

Living with uncertainty

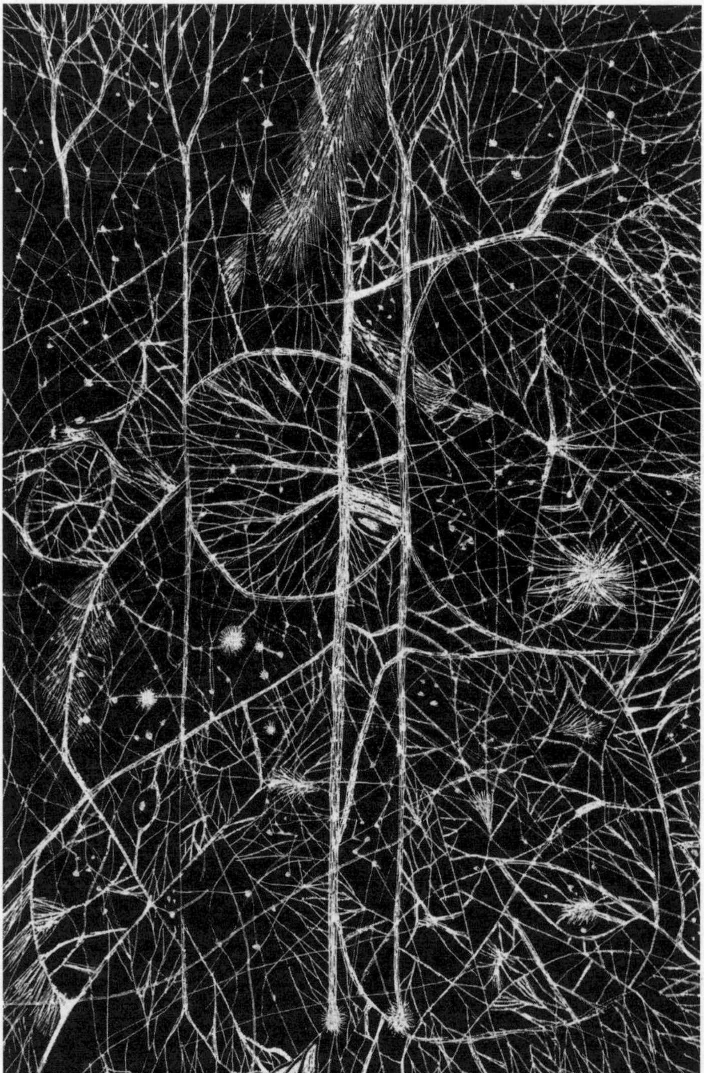

A frequently encountered criticism of psychiatry, and implicitly a way of differentiating psychiatry from general medicine, is its incertitude. With this comes a range of assumptions – that psychiatry is vague and therefore unscientific; that, in comparison to general medicine, its basic tenets are ill-understood; and, possibly as a consequence of this, that its treatments are ineffective. According to this scenario, general medicine progresses triumphantly and seamlessly. If there are uncertainties, these are expected soon to be dispelled by the inexorable forward march of biomedical science. This dichotomous way of thinking is entrenched in medical school training, the institutions of medicine, the separation of psychiatry from other specialities, and modern, materialist, cultural ways of thinking.

Psychiatry is about the mind, and since there is no clear understanding about what might constitute the mind, psychiatry is uncertain. It is a 'Cinderella' discipline. In the popular imagination, it quite possibly belongs more to early-twentieth-century central Europe than the twenty-first century. For many, the ridiculous image still prevails of the psychiatrist as a middle-aged man with a beard, sitting at the head of a couch taking notes, while a younger middle-class woman lies turned away from him, rambling on interminably about her dreams and her sexual fantasies.

This dualist way of thinking – this separation of mind and body, of the psychological and the physical, formalised in the separation of psychiatry from general medicine – is not helpful, has no basis in contemporary neuroscience and is probably harmful. Defining a problem as psychiatric leads to the neglect of physical aspects of the presenting problem and is all too often perceived as dismissive. 'It's all in the mind' is interpreted as 'it's not real'. Conversely, defining a problem as physical leads to the neglect of important psychological factors that require attention. Depression might be a manifestation of a neuroendocrine problem. Being unaware of the likelihood of a person living with a terminal cancer being depressed seems cruelly reductive, unimaginative and unhelpful. The status of the dementias is unclear. The symptoms, certainly in the early stages, are psychological and the biological basis of the process is fairly well elucidated. This group of disorders seems to be both psychiatric and medical. With the rapidly developing understanding of the biological basis of the schizophrenia spectrum disorders, this group is increasingly being described as 'neuropsychiatric' in nature. The duality does not seem to hold.

While I was working in a community clinic, a young woman was referred to me by the medical officer working in an adjacent office. The referral note was absurdly brief: 'Known psychiatric patient. Now complains of headache. Please take over management.'

I asked this young woman to clarify what the problem was. She looked at me vaguely and then her head sank to the desk where we were both sitting. She was fortunately accompanied by her mother who told me that her daughter had been perfectly well until three days ago. She had then suffered the sudden onset of a severe headache. It was described as a blow to the back of the head. She had later become drowsy during the day, was agitated at night, and more recently had begun to vomit. The headache had got steadily worse. This was not a psychiatric problem. This was a medical emergency. She was showing features of raised intracranial pressure, in this context most likely to be due to an intracerebral bleed. She needed an urgent CT scan, not the attention of a psychiatrist.

This encounter raises many issues, one being the discrimination so often observed against patients with psychiatric disorders. Having a mental illness somehow disembodies one. Symptoms are without justification attributed to the psychiatric problem. A proper history is not taken. The necessary examination is not performed. The problem is not taken seriously. This has dangerous, possibly life-threatening, consequences.

The medical officer appeared to have been certain that the symptoms were not due to a medical condition, but to the unspecified psychiatric disorder of which a cursory mention had been made. This is inferred because the necessary history and examination had not been undertaken to justify the diagnosis, which was not a diagnosis but a careless assumption. In clinical medicine, certitude requires great caution. Making such assumptions is rarely feasible and it is hazardous.

The discipline of psychiatry is uncertain, but so is general medicine and so is science. I studied for a Bachelor of Arts degree before I started medicine. In our seminars in the arts faculty, we were encouraged to question, to reflect and analyse. There were few facts and even this was open to debate. Is James Joyce's *Ulysses* a good book? Why is it important? Why do we study one text and not another? We gained some rudimentary tools for thinking critically, or at least that was the aim of our teachers. For these reasons, and many others, starting medicine was a struggle for me. I perhaps naïvely transferred this critical way of thinking to the basic sciences. How do we know? How can we be certain of this when we know that what in the past was considered certain has subsequently been proven to be false? I must have been a very irritating and exasperating student, and I was not helping myself, but I did develop the rather vague notion that medicine represented another culture and that it required a different way of thinking. I coped, somehow, but the feeling of not being sure about being sure persisted.

As junior doctors, a most difficult and miserable task was to impart bad news to patients and their families. I cannot remember ever having been told how to do this. 'It is cancer. It is advanced. It is inoperable. There is nothing more that can be done.' Inevitably, the question follows as to how much time is left. I had no idea, of course; nor, it transpired, did many of my seniors at the time, or not with any degree of certainty. We did not have an opportunity to discuss these important issues at any meaningful level but I did form the impression then that a confident, authoritative posture was recommended. A professional certitude was, for some unknown reason, assumed to be more reassuring and consoling than an admission of incertitude. Not being certain became associated with not knowing, or not knowing for sure, and this seemed to be considered unprofessional or merely incompetent.

I have been prescribed statins by my general practitioner because of high cholesterol and a family history of cardiovascular disease. A study was recently published concerning the benefits of statins in preventing cardiac events, or deaths due to heart attacks. Two respected daily newspapers reported the findings. One declared that millions were taking statins unnecessarily, the other that every male over the age of sixty should be taking them. Two very different conclusions were drawn from the same study. Despite the most strenuous and skilled endeavours to define them, the benefits of statins remain unclear. Furthermore, there are drawbacks to taking this preventative medication, including not only the side-effects. The act of taking the statin is a constant reminder of one's vulnerability. With the swallowing of each wretched tablet, the bell tolls of an assured mortality.

Obesity in prosperous and lower- and middle-income countries is a cause for concern, yet the factors that contribute to this and what to do about it remain uncertain. Smoking causes cancer, but it is not that straightforward. Person A smokes forty cigarettes a day for most of his adult life and dies in his eighties of unrelated causes. Person B, who smokes the same amount, is dead as a result of a bronchogenic carcinoma at the age of fifty. How to treat a relatively benign prostatic cancer in an otherwise healthy seventy-year-old man is uncertain. The benefits of surgery for lower back pain are uncertain. Clinical medicine is fraught with uncertainties. The more we seem to know, the more we do not know – or the uncertainties move to another level. An ischaemic event or a heart attack owing to a thrombosis in a coronary artery appears to be fairly clear; the many interacting genetic and environmental factors that contribute to the formation of the thrombosis are much less certain.

For many years, I was required to present an update of research in the field of schizophrenia to the department's weekly journal club. This became challenging. Every year in the literature there was a familiar refrain. These were exciting times. We were on the verge of discovering the causes of schizophrenia. Ten, forty, then over a hundred genes were identified as being contributory. The expectation was that with the elucidation of the causes more effective treatments would become possible. This has not happened, or whether it has happened or not is open to debate. It is by no means certain. After so many years, after so many endeavours and so many millions of dollars spent on research, the causes of schizophrenia and an effective remedy for it remain elusive.

Some time ago, I probably annoyed my colleagues by presenting an image of a half-filled glass and saying that, with regard to schizophrenia research, I was not sure whether the glass was half-full or half-empty. I don't think this has changed significantly, which does not mean that research is going nowhere or that the pursuit of the causes of schizophrenia has been futile. It is just more complex than had perhaps been thought, and with complexity comes uncertainty.

The history of science is replete with ideas and beliefs that at the time were held to be certain and in retrospect have been proven false and absurd and even embarrassing. On a visit with colleagues to see a new hospital in Kimberley in the Northern Cape we were given a tour of the Big Hole, a massive excavation pit. A brochure informed us that the most eminent geologist of the time had been tasked by the colonial government to survey the area for possible diamond deposits. After doubtlessly extremely thorough investigations he declared with great certainty that no diamonds were to be found in the area. Within five years the most extensive diamond deposits in the world were discovered at the site. Incidentally, the geologist – apparently undeterred – then formulated an ostrich hypothesis. He had not in fact been mistaken. Ostriches in a distant diamond-rich area had swallowed the diamonds and, moving to Kimberley, had chosen to defecate the precious stones there on a massive and very generous scale.

Uncertainty is not confined to clinical medicine or psychiatry but appears to be an integral aspect of basic science. The very fabric of reality is uncertain. Uncertainty is intrinsic to quantum physics. The nature and extent of dark matter and dark energy are not known, nor is it clear why matter should be, rather than there being nothing. It does not seem to be known whether we inhabit a universe or a multiverse. Why time should have a direction, and the origins and the ultimate fate of the universe or multiverse, are profound mysteries. The world is made up of matter and force and particles comprising, we are informed, a deeply mysterious web of fermions, up-and-down quarks and bosons. That is where things are for the time being, it seems, but in a discussion with a young physicist recently he told me that there was uncertainty in his circles about what might actually constitute a particle, or whether a particle might perhaps be a length of string or a wave.

Uncertainty does not have to be a problem. It can be a source of wonder. It is a driving force for answering important questions, for solving mysteries. Certainties can be oppressive. There is no further to go. Doors close. The problem perhaps has more to do with how we live with uncertainty – as if, in some way, to survive we need to believe in some things being certain, however illusory that might be.

A vastly complex array of factors contribute to acts of terror but one possibly neglected factor might be the yearning, independent of religion, for certitude. The modern world is too complex and too various. It is not possible to reconcile this alien world with the teachings of the ancient texts. Values are no longer absolute but relative, in a way that is bewildering and contradictory. A fundamentalist position represents more solid ground. The notion of fundamentalism itself is fraught with uncertainty but one aspect would seem to be an inclination to interpret the texts in a more concrete way, a disinclination to tolerance and, as a consequence, a higher risk of seeking transcendence in the rapture of oblivion and martyrdom.

Perhaps the most personal and existential uncertainty of our lives is when and how we will die. Most of us prefer to live with this uncertainty but that we get older rather than younger is certain, as is the fact of our mortality. Even this, however, is disputed by some of our more technologically inclined fellow beings who imagine and plan to defeat death by having themselves, whatever those selves might be, frozen or uploaded to the cloud. Yet there is no escaping incertitude: it is unknown whether this disembodied software might or might not be a desirable state of being.

Given the positive nature of incertitude, of not knowing propelling us forward to knowing, it seems that we nevertheless have to come to terms with the very human unease of having to live with inevitable uncertainty. Certainties are consoling. We comfort children, we seek to persuade ourselves that the world is a secure place, that there are landmarks and signposts and beacons that will reliably guide us on our way. We are not inclined to contemplate the chaos of the universe.

We seek patterns or shapes of meaning in order to make predictions so that we can plan, and hopefully gain some degree of control over our lives. It is a tentative process. Living with uncertainty is discomforting but being in a world that is entirely certain is unimaginable. It is also hazardous, inducing an inertia that may undermine the seeking necessary for survival. A total certainty or predictability would make our lives empty and devoid of any need to make choices or take action. A paralysis of boredom induced by the illusion of certitude seems an undesirable state of mind or being.

It is a matter of finding some balance between a degree of predictability in order to cope as best we can, and accepting – but not being overwhelmed by – uncertainty. This all goes to pieces in psychotic states. There is no balance.

The parents of Rudewaan listen to me anxiously. He has recently been admitted to our unit and I don't think there can be any doubt that the diagnosis is schizophrenia. 'But Doctor, how can you be sure?' 'How long will it take for him to get better?' 'Will he get better?' 'Will he be able to work?' 'Will he be himself again?' 'Will he be able to lead a normal life, study, work, marry, have children, look after us when we get old?' These questions get asked again and again, and I wish I could answer them with certainty, but I know it would be unjustified. I am the consultant. I am the senior doctor in the unit. There is nowhere else for the family to turn for the answers they so understandably need. It is difficult to accept the diagnosis of schizophrenia, and all the more difficult to come to terms with the many uncertainties that such a diagnosis entails.

I try to explain the problem to the students. We attempt a discussion of what constitutes a diagnosis. The diagnosis of tuberculosis is not the same as a diagnosis of schizophrenia. I talk of a 'tentative, provisional hypothesis', and it is clear that they are dissatisfied. Science is to do with facts, with certitudes. Therein lies its great successes, and that is unquestionable. Without the solid basis of empirical, objective, verifiable, factual information, the status of biomedical science becomes tenuous. The inclination to certitude is understandable and leads to a growing confidence and the proud claim of being a professional. Doubt is difficult. It gets in the way. It is messy but necessary.

Finding the balance is often difficult, and the boundaries shift. It is not helpful to anybody, not to patients nor families nor practitioners, to wallow in a sea of uncertainty and doubt and confusion. It is also not helpful to adopt a position of confident certainty when the circumstances do not allow it. Some things are inevitably uncertain, some things less so; sometimes it is appropriate to be certain and sometimes it is not.

Attitudes and styles of performing also change with time, and the practice of medicine is subject to cultural shifts. Generalisations are to be avoided, and I am not sure if this might have been due to my lowly position as a medical student but I do have the impression that the consultants when I was a student were more arrogant. They seemed to be more unquestionably certain of their superior knowledge and their unfailing capacity to solve whichever challenging problems they encountered. They were often referred to ironically as gods and often they behaved like gods, being literally minded. I don't think it's like that any longer, or certainly not to such an extent. Why this should be so is yet another uncertainty. It does seem plausible that the sheer accumulation of information has had a paradoxically humbling effect, that such hubris is inappropriate – and certainly that knowing everything is impossible.

5

The boundaries of mental illness and the problems of living

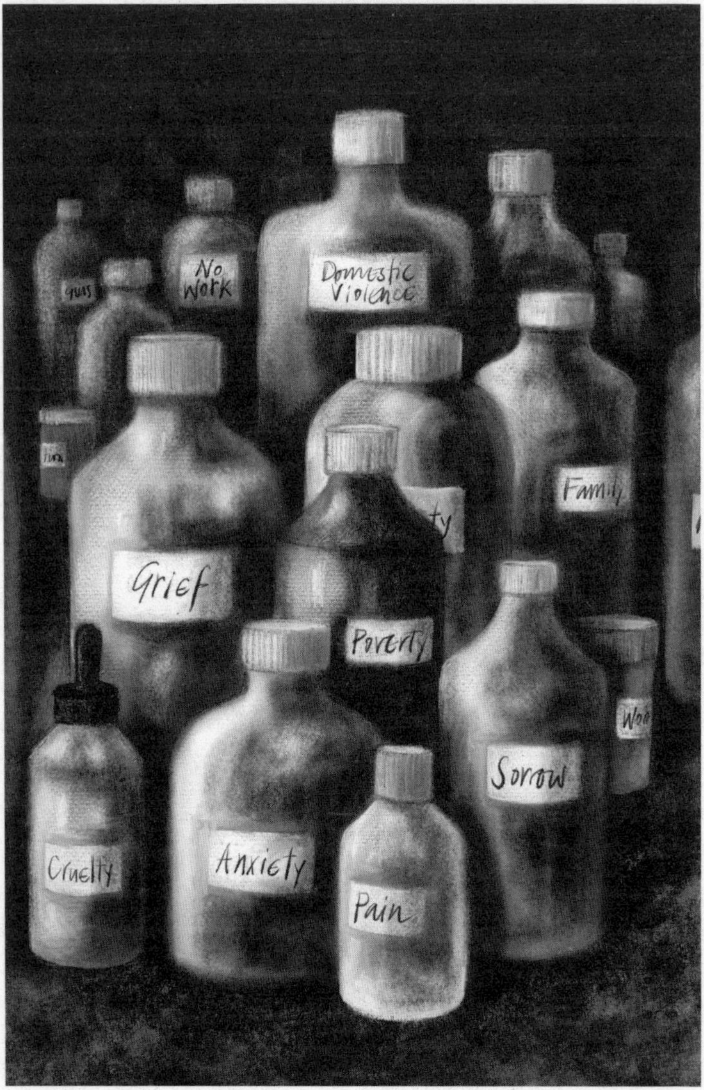

The boundaries of mental illness are overextended. A number of factors contribute to this fairly recent phenomenon. One driving force is a reaction to the relative neglect of mental illness in the past and a concomitant lack of funding for research into the causes and effective treatment of these disorders. To emphasise the prevalence and the burden of mental illness a claim is made that one in five adults in the general population will, at some stage of their lives, suffer from some form of mental disorder. It is not clear whether such a claim furthers understanding and reduces stigma, or is unhelpful and potentially harmful.

One aspect of possible harm is that, given such a broad definition of what might constitute illness, the claim will be dismissed as a misrepresentation of the problems of living as symptoms of a mental disorder. The *Diagnostic and Statistical Manual of Mental Disorders* (DSM-5) published by the American Psychiatric Association has been dramatically expanded. Problems such as bereavement disorder and oppositional defiant disorder are included, raising concerns as to whether these are new, meaningful categories, and whether invoking the notion of a disorder in this respect is helpful – or might instead undermine coping strategies. Diagnosed as suffering from a mental illness, a bereaved person might understandably be more inclined to resort to medication than seek the support of family and friends.

The great majority of the mental disorders in this twenty per cent of the general adult population constitute anxiety and depressive disorders. The problem arises as to what might be considered a valid, reliable threshold for making such diagnoses. Anxiety and depression are problems of living. These difficult – at times, deeply unpleasant and agonising – emotional states prompt responses that can be, and probably are for the most part, beneficial. Understanding and support are enlisted. The intensity and the incapacity also tend to pass with time. A diagnosis of mental illness is more likely to slow the process and confound strategies for recovery. How one copes with suffering is a question of values, and there should be great caution in prescribing how one should do so. Problems arise when scientific attitudes intrude with claims of objectivity and a panoply of operationally defined diagnostic guidelines.

The difficulties posed by boundaries or thresholds also pertain to the rather arbitrary distinction between serious and other mental illnesses. Schizophrenia, bipolar disorders and the most severe depressive disorders generally fall into the 'serious' category. Most anxiety and depressive disorders do not, and it is this group that accounts for the escalating worldwide diagnoses of mental illness. How 'other' mental illnesses, as opposed to 'serious' ones, are defined is not made explicit, but 'unserious' or 'not so serious' is surely implicit. It is difficult to imagine someone in the throes of an anxiety attack or in the anguish of a depression not being enraged by such apparent disregard. The notion of a 'not serious' or 'not severe' illness is ridiculous, and raises the question of why it should be considered an illness at all – and what purpose there might be in invoking illness or a pathological process other than to profit the pharmaceutical industry.

Further problems arise with regard to the allocation of limited resources and to appropriate management. An argument is made that the expansion of the diagnoses of anxiety and depression diverts attention and resources away from schizophrenia and bipolar disorders, representing greater burdens in terms of disability and suffering. This is disputed, and depression is estimated to be one of the major causes of disability in the near future. A diagnosis implies the need for treatment. This raises further difficulties in that it is not clear what are the most appropriate and effective treatments for anxiety and depression. Controversies abound as to whether medication or various forms of psychotherapy or a combination of these is more appropriate, and the matter is further confounded by some evidence that treatment of whatever nature is less effective for these disorders than for the more serious forms of mental illness, given the inadequacy of this term. It stands to some reason that grief will not be diminished by either a diagnosis or an antidepressant.

There are lethal consequences to this possibly rather abstract notion of definitions and boundaries and thresholds. At the time of writing, concern is rising in the USA about an epidemic of opioid addiction. Deaths from overdose are similar in number to those caused by motor-vehicle accidents. Opioids are among the most common causes of mortality in those under fifty. Opioids are also big business. Opioid painkillers generate billions of dollars in sales, as do treatment programmes for addiction and overdoses. It seems doubtful that the escalation in the prescription of opioids corresponds directly to a recent rise in the phenomenon of pain. It is more probable that the escalation is in the diagnosis of a pain disorder, considered to warrant this potentially lethal treatment. Of course, the problem is compounded by misuse, abuse and addiction, but the opioids are prescribed initially mostly as appropriate and effective treatments for pain.

Opioids are effective treatments for acute pain, much less so for chronic pain, which far outweighs acute pain as an indication for treatment. Opioids for the treatment of chronic pain are of doubtful efficacy and are clearly dangerous. It follows that the diagnosis of a chronic pain syndrome has potentially hazardous consequences – and that, for this reason, the validity and the utility of the diagnosis must be carefully scrutinised. For the most part, a diagnosis is probably not made, and the presentation of the symptoms of pain is considered sufficient justification for the prescription of an opioid.

Pain is a universal phenomenon that has value in protecting the body from actual or potential harm. In its chronic form, it is without value. It is an expression of suffering, and in this respect may be considered to be a problem of living. The translation of chronic pain into a medical problem with a medical solution is too often unhelpful – and harmful.

I met Magda only once, in a busy community clinic on the outskirts of the city. The complaint had been of widespread pain. This had become steadily worse over the previous six months, and was becoming intolerable. She had been examined by the medical officer, who could find nothing to account for her symptoms. The referral note was brief, and indicated that in the absence of any physical findings the problem must be of a psychiatric nature. No mention was made of even a cursory mental-state examination to support this conclusion.

She recounted a story of many misfortunes and seemingly insoluble problems. After years of abuse she had eventually been deserted by her drunken husband. She had no work and was in dire financial straits. Her teenage daughter was pregnant and she was sure that her son was abusing drugs. He had dropped out of school. She felt desperate and did not know where to turn. She was exhausted all the time and her body ached. I told her I thought she was suffering, that her body was feeling it, that it was all too much. She seemed relieved by this.

'Yes. Yes,' she said. '*Dit is my senuwees, Dokter.*' (It is my nerves, Doctor.)

She sought an explanation, not a diagnosis. There was no evidence of a medical problem nor of a psychiatric disorder. She did not need to be told that there was anything wrong with her. This was more likely to make her feel worse and further undermine her very limited resources. She was struggling, certainly. Her pain was understandable. Her suffering needed to be acknowledged. She was not depressed and not unduly anxious. There was no need for medication nor any particular form of counselling other than for me to register and acknowledge her predicament.

Clinicians often describe being under pressure to make a diagnosis and to prescribe medication, and often admit to an unease about this, recognising that they do not believe it will do any good but feeling a need to do something. With regard to Magda, this seemed more likely to be interpreted as a paternalistic dismissal of the extent and gravity of her problems. These actions are not neutral and not without consequences. Problems of living are transformed into medical or psychiatric problems, and are then treated in a way that is not helpful and is all the more likely to lead to a perception of not being in control; thence, a downward spiral to helplessness. This woman was proud. She was dignified. Her circumstances were dire and unjust, but she was not in any way broken. She needed to be respected. Being a doctor, it seemed important to me then not to be a doctor.

In circumstances such as these, the diagnoses of fibromyalgia or chronic fatigue syndrome or myalgic encephalomyelitis are often invoked. This is the language of medicine, of pathology, and the terms are most commonly used in the specialist domains of neurology and rheumatology. In psychiatry, the categories of somatoform disorders, or somatic symptom disorders, or medically unexplained symptoms, are more likely to be used, and all are unsatisfactory. Somatoform disorders or somatic symptom disorders are unhelpful because the terms indicate a psychiatric disorder that many presenting with such symptoms would understandably find offensive, interpreting this as dismissive; and 'medically unexplained symptoms' is an unsatisfactory term because it is unexplained. These terms are also problematic in that there is no evidence to support a diagnosis of encephalomyelitis or the rather arbitrarily defined fibromyalgia – if objectively verifiable biological pathologies are considered necessary for such alarming-sounding diagnoses to be made, rather than the symptoms of pain and fatigue.

Sebastian described a range of shifting emotions and thoughts and behaviours after his father, to whom he had been very close, had died suddenly and unexpectedly.

'From the start I cannot remember the feelings, specifically of grief. I was more confused or disoriented. It seemed to be a different world. Things that were meaningful or important changed. Light and colour drained away. I don't think I cared very much about anything any longer. I did not think about the future. I didn't think I would be part of it. I didn't care very much about myself. I don't think I was self-destructive, but certainly, looking back, I took stupid risks. Life was empty. It seemed to be a charade. I did not care very much if I was alive or dead. Then, very slowly, colour and texture in the smallest detail began to emerge in my world. Cautiously, I retrieved meaning and purpose in life. I became engaged in work, marriage and children. I have not forgotten the loss, of course. It will always be part of my life, and I suppose I would not be whoever I am without what has happened to me. That goes for all of us, surely. Somehow we find a way of going on. I can't compare my experience with others but things are possibly now more intense, or precious and vivid.'

Sebastian did not seek a diagnosis. He did not think that there was anything wrong with him. He did not consider that a diagnosis would in some way affirm his struggle to cope with the death of his father. He regarded the struggle as something inevitable and believed that the symptoms he interpreted in the context of mourning would pass with time. A diagnosis of a bereavement disorder in this circumstance seems wrong and unhelpful and invalidating, and an insult to one's efforts to cope with adversity.

Intrinsic to the notion of a diagnosis or the construct of some form of disorder, whether psychiatric or not, is the expectation of a cure or a solution. A clinician might seek to qualify this and claim that for many disorders the belief in a cure is inappropriate – and that effective management might be the best that can be hoped for. This may be so, but in the lay imagination the provision of some form of cure is what follows from a provision of a diagnosis. The symptom is identified and treated with the assumption that it is then eliminated. The problem is solved and the person who is no longer a patient gets on with his or her life. But loss is not something that can be solved. The hardship and social and economic adversity contributing to the symptoms of pain and fatigue are not going to go away, and to allow that this might not be so with the provision of what is called treatment is simplistic and patronising and mendacious.

The pharmaceutical industry might profit, but among members of the general, more critically minded population the response to this process of pathologising problems of living is likely to be scepticism and cynicism and an increasing disenchantment with modern medicine. This phenomenon is as evident in general medicine as it is in psychiatry, and is reflected in a trend towards alternative or complementary forms of medicine.

This is no simple answer – but psychiatry is not furthering its cause by reaching beyond its limits.

6

The confounding limits of science

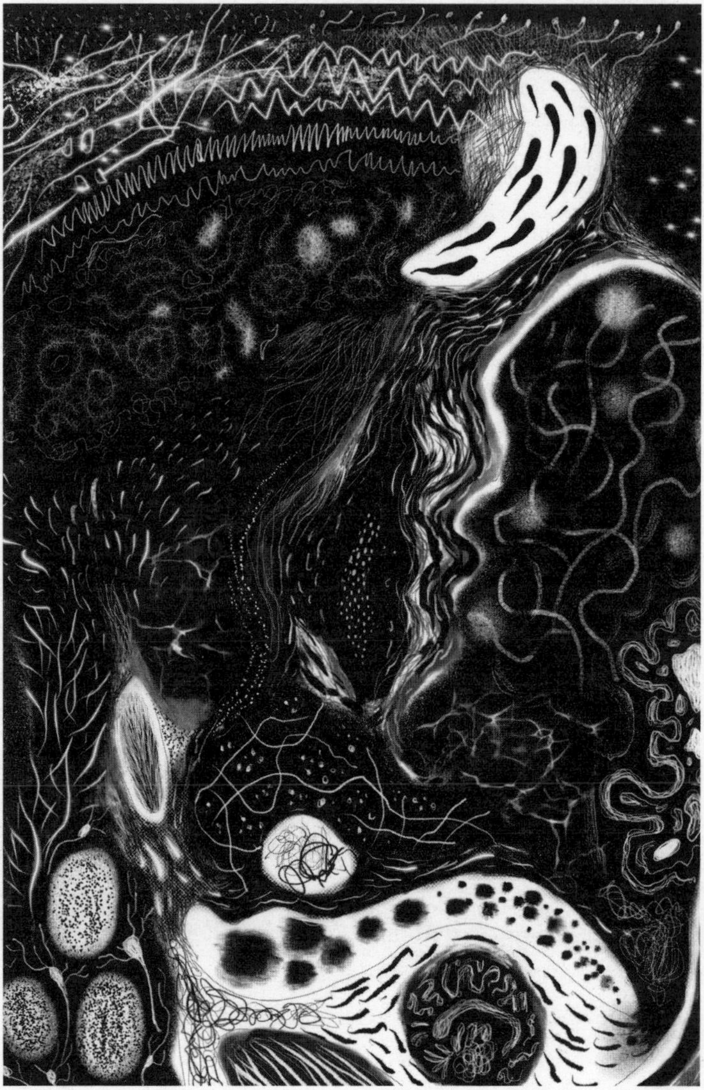

'I feel they want to know about me … they want to influence me detrimentally … they want to know what I am doing in the breathing world … I go under attack from the outside world … people affect me … my pulse … my heart beating … my breathing …'

'I could not take it any more … he was making me crazy … I had to throttle him … the voices were telling me to shut him up … he is the king of calamity … I am the king of peace …'

'I am Jeremiah … I am Allah … I am responsible for the downfall of mankind … I am deaf … I am blind … I am being punished for the Fall … but I said Eve don't do it … Eve! Don't eat the banana! But she ate the banana, and now I am punished … and we are doomed …'

What these idiosyncratic utterances have to do with the neurobiological basis of schizophrenia is a mystery. Dopamine dysregulation, or a fault in the expression of an array of interacting genetic variants, or a dysconnectivity of neuronal networks in the higher centres of the brain, cannot explain the strangeness and the anguish implicit in these accounts. Nor is any common denominator evident, which might be expected if there is a shared pathophysiology, other than distress and a sense of threat and injustice. This disjunction reflects a deep and ancient philosophical problem, and so should not surprise us. How mind arises from the matter of the brain is an enduring and enigmatic problem.

Psychiatry concerns itself with disorders of the mind and claims to be a scientific discipline. Definitions of what constitutes the conscious mind are various, but include notions of subjectivity, intentionality, agency and autonomy. Subjectivity is integral to the concept of mind, and the feeling of who we are and what we are not. A problem then arises as to how to provide a scientific account of the mind and its maladies, if central to the scientific method is a requirement of objectivity.

An indication of the scientific aspiration is the development of operationally defined diagnostic systems in psychiatry. Schizophrenia is defined by a set of rules. For example, delusions and hallucinations and some degree of functional impairment must be evident and the symptoms should not be accounted for by a general medical condition or substance abuse. These rules are explicit and objectively verifiable. The diagnostic process, therefore, in terms of a degree of reliability meets basic scientific criteria. This does represent progress in that the diagnosis of schizophrenia, with all its potentially damaging implications, is not left to mere intuition – or, as I was taught in my undergraduate years, 'a feeling'.

I remember the professor imparting this to us by waving his fingers in the air in a vague fluttering motion, as if to communicate the inadequacy of words. I recall being frustrated: this did not conform to my youthful notions of scientific rigour. But in retrospect he was perhaps saying or suggesting something important that has become lost in a triumphalist belief in scientific progress. Then, we believed in some vague way that it was just a matter of time – that soon the cause of schizophrenia would be discovered, and with the known cause would come the cure. The reliability of the diagnosis was, at least, the first step.

A number of problems have arisen in this regard that have placed limitations on such optimism. Schizophrenia has come to be regarded less as a provisional, hypothetical construct than a thing out there, an object of scientific enquiry. The subjective dimension, which is surely central to any study of the mind and its disorders, is marginalised or neglected.

Related to this is an uncertainty regarding the diagnostic validity of such a reified construct. Schizophrenia is not a thing that can be measured or verified by some validating objective marker. To this day, and confounding the expectations of the past, there is no genetic test or neuroimaging study that can confirm the presence or absence of schizophrenia. In another language, whether or not a person is suffering from schizophrenia is beyond the realm of science. Suffering is not amenable to measurement.

It would be absurd to seek to estimate the quantum of suffering appropriate for a broken leg or a broken heart.

The question also arises as to whether the term 'schizophrenia' can provide an adequate or meaningful account of the protean expressions of the disorder – and whether such an abstract formulation problematically neglects schizophrenia's phenomenology, or the lived experience of schizophrenia. There is a tension between objective, verifiable, third-person accounts of mental states and subjective, deeply personal, first-person accounts. To develop an adequate and useful understanding and explanation of the problem of schizophrenia neither perspective can be put aside. The objective and subjective positions are not binary opposites but complementary. Coming to some basic and useful understanding of psychotic phenomena must incorporate first-person accounts, however difficult, incoherent and obscure these might be. Dismissing these phenomena simply because personal perspectives fail to meet the conventional criteria for scientific objectivity limits understanding and lacks the rigour and comprehensiveness that is surely an important part of the scientific method.

In current standard practice, there is a gulf between diagnostic explanation and a sufficient understanding of the predicament of an individual in a specific personal, social and cultural context. This reaches beyond the confines of psychiatry. It is a frequently heard complaint in general medicine that one is treated merely as an object by a harried clinician, a mere assembly of symptoms. It is difficult to imagine how the fear of an early death can be separated from a diagnosis of cancer, or how an abusive partner or socioeconomic deprivation or grave personal loss might be considered irrelevant to a complaint of chronic pain and fatigue.

An adequate understanding – for example, of the phenomena of schizophrenia – is lacking. Such an understanding would require at least some degree of integration of three levels: the neurobiological deficits or derangements; the cognitive and emotional correlates; and the subjective experience of these aberrant processes. It would not be helpful – and it would have grave implications for the pharmacological treatment of schizophrenia – if, for example, we chose to associate delusions with diminished rather than increased dopamine transmission, or vice versa with regard to problems of executive function. We would be aggravating, not alleviating, the problem. Psychotic symptoms are not simply eliminated by antipsychotic medications. We need a more nuanced and precise definition of the nature of the psychotic symptoms.

Diagnostic explanation and meaningful understanding need to be integrated into clinical practice and research programmes – to foster an improved therapeutic alliance and to clarify the neurobiological basis for specific symptoms rather than overarching disease categories. To ask what meanings might be attached to symptoms such as hearing voices is not to be nice and polite, or culturally sensitive. Doing so might, among many other things, guide us as to whether any form of intervention is warranted in the first place. Focusing on specific symptoms rather than broader diagnostic constructs might also guide us towards more precise and valid neurobiological correlates.

Related to the uncertainties regarding the validity of psychiatric diagnoses are the arbitrariness of many operationally defined criteria, the considerable overlap between diagnostic categories and the very indistinct boundaries between mental illness and what might be considered to be within the bounds of non-pathological human experience. This applies most obviously to problems such as anxiety and depression, but extends also to psychotic phenomena. There is a debate as to whether psychosis should be most appropriately regarded as a category or a dimension. This, again, seems to be caught up in the tensions between the requirements of validity and reliability. Reliability favours a categorical formulation: understanding psychosis in dimensional terms might be a more valid approach but eludes reliable determination.

The trend towards understanding psychotic phenomena on a

spectrum has been given impetus in recent years by the attention paid to the prevalence of psychotic experiences in the general, relatively healthy population. Many people simply find ways of coping with psychotic symptoms. Various strategies might be adopted, very probably including granting meaning to these idiosyncratic experiences and embedding the phenomena in personal and cultural contexts. These can be effective ways of alleviating the distress associated with an experience that might otherwise be further complicated and aggravated by being perceived as pathological. It is bad enough believing that others want to do you harm; this is made worse by being told you are sick or mad.

Possibly enabled by Facebook, a young man in the outpatient clinic told me of hearing voices asking him if they could be his 'friend'. These voices were not perceived as malicious or pathological. They were consoling to him. There was no reason to take them away. In another context, a young man appeared to be reassured that the voices he heard were communications from his ancestors.

Merely defining these experiences as auditory hallucinations seems restricted. The meanings attached to the experience are more likely to be more important to the person than the definition of psychopathology. This is of concern because it determines what form of intervention should be made, if any, and this has ethical ramifications. There is an important difference between paternalism and a more respectful, collaborative way of trying to help people living with psychotic experiences. It is less the symptom itself than the distress and the impairments it might engender that is of concern. In an ideal world, and if a degree of insight is retained, it is then for the person who is experiencing psychotic symptoms to decide if help is needed and what form that help should take. The assumption that psychotic phenomena are inherently pathological and should therefore be suppressed needs to be reconsidered.

Another assumption underlying the way in which psychosis is understood, and consequently treated, is the notion that there is a fault in the way in which a person with psychosis perceives the external world in contrast to the more accurate appraisal of the world by those not affected by psychosis. This rather simplistic distinction is called into question by current neurocognitive formulations of how the world is perceived and enters into our consciousness. It is evident that sensory signals are relatively crude or elemental, and that a time lag exists between the activation of receptors and the entry of these signals into our consciousness. Perceptions in this regard are conceptualised as inferences or beliefs about the world. I see what I believe, rather than I believe what I see.

These rather abstract considerations do have implications for how we imagine and treat severe mental illnesses. Symptoms of psychosis are constructions not dissimilar to the way in which we all try to make sense of the world, and in the context of psychosis may be understood as attempts to give some form to what might otherwise be experienced as intolerable noise. These endeavours then need, in some way, to be acknowledged rather than eliminated or merely neglected. Modulation of salience, limiting distress and enhancing the capacity to cope might be more helpful and appropriate goals of treatment than the suppression of experiences that are desperately real for those who have them.

The fundamental pathophysiological deficits and the ultimate causes of the syndrome of schizophrenia remain unknown. Looking beyond the signs and the symptoms, attending to the experience of psychosis, and linking this to observable phenomena and known neurobiological shifts may yield more meaningful results and more valid diagnostic constructs. First- and third-person perspectives need to be integrated if advances are to be made. The rigid implementation of reductive scientific models has generated a bland and bleak depiction of psychosis that does not accord with the strange and extraordinary stories we encounter in our wards.

The limits are especially confounding because, in contrast to other fields of scientific endeavour, little progress seems to have been made in the field of mental illness – and in schizophrenia in particular. This might be disputed, but in my experience the expectations at the time when I was beginning my career in psychiatry have not been realised. There are many possible reasons for this. As the human brain is the most complicated thing in the known universe, however, this observation should not be surprising. Related to this is the notion that the human brain does not have the capacity to understand itself or the nature of consciousness. An argument could then be made that it is merely a matter of time, and that with the rapid development of artificial intelligence, this obstacle will be overcome. A smart machine will solve the problem.

A further conundrum then arises in that if we do not have the intellectual capacity as humans to know the nature of ourselves, it is unclear how we will be able to know that our brains have been superseded. We will not have the intelligence to grasp that there is an intelligence superior to our own. If that might be so, it is uncertain how we might be able to use the information derived from this superior intelligence in an intelligent and useful way. Another difficulty lies in the order of investigation. It is curious that we should imagine that we can begin to understand how things go wrong when we do not understand how they work in the first place.

We might begin, then, by seeking to understand what it means to feel that you are under attack from the outside world, that voices are compelling you to throttle the king of calamity, or that you are responsible for the fall of mankind and are therefore doomed. I do not think these utterances are without meaning. Choosing to believe that the psychotic experience is of no relevance within the confines of a biomedical framework limits our capacity to be helpful.

7
The biology of madness

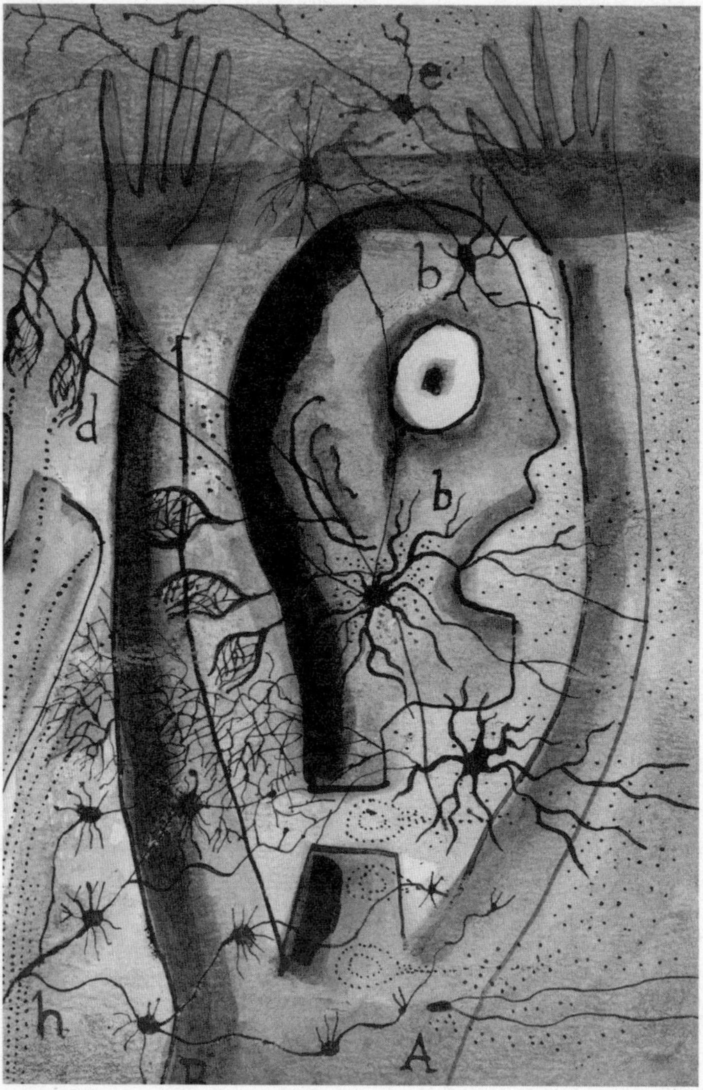

There are two universities with medical faculties in the Western Cape. They are approximately fifty kilometres apart, but traditionally are culturally, historically and politically distinct. Both faculties have departments of psychiatry. For much of the time while I was a student, and until quite recently, these departments held different – and, at times, opposing – positions with regard to the nature and causes of mental illness.

The one department was considered to be 'biological' in orientation. Mental illness was caused by an array of biological factors and in this respect a 'biomedical model' was considered most appropriate. This required the identification of a number of specified signs and symptoms for a diagnosis to be made. The predominant form of treatment was medication, intended to treat the biological factors that were presumed to be the causes of the illness characterised by the specific diagnosis. This was more or less in line with a European way of thinking about psychiatry. Psychiatry was a medical speciality. The as-yet-undetermined causes of mental illness were presumed to be biological, and therefore the treatment was essentially physical.

At the adjacent institution, on the other side of the river, an alternative way of thinking prevailed. Mental illnesses were of a fundamentally psychological nature. The causes were due to psychological conflict, often arising from childhood experiences. These conflicts were for the most part of an unconscious nature, and treatment involved bringing these repressed events to the surface – with the assumption that in this clear light of consciousness the symptoms would resolve. Not much attention was paid to making diagnoses. Of greater interest were the psychological processes giving rise to the presenting problems. This position was more aligned to a predominantly American psychoanalytical tradition. Treatment was therefore of a more psychotherapeutic nature, and there was much less emphasis and interest in physical treatments. Psychiatry was not really a science. It occupied an uncertain space between medicine and the humanities.

Partly as a consequence of these divergent positions, the one department had a much stronger tradition of research than the other. Viewing the phenomena of mental illness objectively enables scientific enquiry. Identifying symptoms according to operationally defined criteria; using rating scales to measure changes, for example, in the mental state in response to one or other medication; and employing randomised, controlled clinical trials to investigate the effectiveness (or not) of various treatments brought psychiatry into alignment with general medicine. Psychiatry should no longer be regarded as a marginal discipline, rather embarrassingly lagging behind the other disciplines in its lack of scientific rigour and compromised by its uncertainties.

Over the past few years these differences have diminished, and possibly withered away altogether. The psychoanalytical tradition has waned in influence, particularly with regard to serious mental illness or the psychoses. This is in all likelihood due to a number of reasons, including rapid advances in the neurosciences – but also, perhaps in an increasingly scientific world, an awkward lack of evidence to support often-extravagant claims and an equally problematic absence of evidence that psychoanalytical treatments are at all effective.

At the time I remember these two different ways of thinking giving rise to a quite teasing, mostly healthy rivalry. The 'biological' position was dismissed as crude and reductionist, the other as non-scientific and vague, and this led to discussions and debates that were for the most part friendly and possibly creative. I do not remember any real antagonism; perhaps this reflected an awareness that this dichotomous way of thinking was false, and far too simplistic a conceptual framework for understanding a fundamental problem implicit in the tension between the two positions. This arises from the persisting and profoundly mysterious relationship between the mind and the brain.

Regardless of current neuroscientific and philosophical thinking, it seems very probable that for many if not most of us there is an unwillingness or a refusal to consider that who we are might arise from mere matter. It is intolerable; it is an affront to believe that our most intimate thoughts, our deepest feelings, our very souls might be mere ephemera, or the epiphenomena of central nervous system electrochemical signalling bound within the absurdly confined limits of the skull.

This disquiet is reflected in debates about what might constitute the nature of mental illness and how it should best be managed. Sometimes this is explicit; more often the assumptions that inform our thinking are implicit. We are uncertain, at some level, about whether madness is an affliction of the brain or the soul – and then about whether it should be treated by a doctor or a priest or a shaman. We might feel squeamish about, or regard as abhorrent, the fact that a psychotropic medication – a tablet that blocks dopamine transmission in certain parts of the brain – should be used to treat the profound perturbations of our souls or our psyches.

The difficulty seems to arise, again, from a dichotomous way of thinking – an unexamined belief that it is one thing or the other, that it is either biological or psychological, reflecting a seventeenth-century dualism that persists to the present. It is very probable that these fundamental philosophical issues underpin many of the debates and controversies in contemporary psychiatry. Yet many of those advocating one position or another would likely doubt the relevance of philosophy to the question of how mental illness should be conceptualised. It seems also less of a scientific issue than a problem of belief or dogma. Over the many years during which I have worked as a psychiatrist, it has been disappointing that these polarities seem to have persisted. This is despite remarkable advances in the understanding of how the brain works, and what happens when it does not work, and – in the philosophical domain – despite advances way beyond the dualism of Descartes, however vexed the question of the nature of consciousness might still be.

The difficulties might arise to some extent from the limitations of science or a scientific way of thinking. Who we are, the way we think and feel and behave, and consequently the nature of the aberrations of these very human faculties are not a matter for scientific investigation. These are issues of belief or of faith. This transcendent and consoling edifice of our notion of ourselves, our humanity, can surely not be reduced to mere matter, the stuff of the brain. It cannot be that this cathedral we imagine of ourselves might just be a precarious construction of bricks and mortar and broken glass.

This is a refusal of the evolution of our species, but also of contemporary thinking in the neurosciences about the complex relationships between mind, brain and the environment. Binary thinking might appear to make things simple, but in all likelihood the issues become more muddled and distorted. Related to the problematic mind–brain dualism is another prevalent question, usually also framed in a dichotomous way, as to whether the causes of mental illness are biological or environmental. The question poses its own problems. A more appropriate enquiry might be to consider the nature of the interaction between biological and environmental factors that give rise to mental illness. The way we think about these matters is further confused by the assumptions we make about causation being linear and unidirectional.

Arno is drinking too much, his wife complains, because he is depressed. He is depressed because he has been fired from his job. He got fired because he was drinking too much. Perhaps he was drinking too much because he was depressed at work. Perhaps the depression was caused by his drinking getting out of control. Perhaps we complicate things for ourselves by trying to see things in linear terms when a rather more messy complex of interacting factors might be a more valid interpretation.

Nemba was admitted to our unit after what appeared to be a long history of gradual deterioration in health, culminating in a dramatic escalation of overtly psychotic symptoms. He had been cared for by his grandmother. The father had reportedly suffered from some form of mental illness. He had abused alcohol and died in a violent altercation when Nemba was six. The father had abused the mother, and possibly as a consequence the mother had herself resorted to a dependency on alcohol. This had eventually led to her death in her early forties. Nemba struggled from the beginning of his life, perhaps understandably in the circumstances. He began to fail at school and was admonished by his teachers for being stupid and mocked by the other children for his odd appearance. He was eventually sent for an assessment, and a diagnosis was made of a mild to moderate intellectual impairment associated with the features of foetal alcohol syndrome. With little or no family or professional support, and with no confidence in himself, Nemba started to avoid classes – and then drifted away from schooling altogether. The grandmother applied for a disability grant on the basis of his intellectual impairment and her application was successful.

In these circumstances, it was almost inevitable that Nemba should become involved in the gangsterism that was rife in the townships. He was extremely vulnerable and the small income he gained from the disability grant was very attractive to the gangsters, who soon exploited his desperate wish to belong by selling him drugs and enlisting him in criminal activities. Things took a miserably predictable course. He drifted downwards, his behaviour became increasingly erratic and disorganised, and eventually the police were called when he threatened his grandmother with violence. He said he would kill her if she did not give him money for drugs. When the police arrived he was raving incoherently; it was apparent to them that he was ill. After three days in the psychiatric unit of the local day hospital there was no change in his behaviour and he was transferred to our hospital.

It is clear that no single cause can be identified to account for this lamentable trajectory, and that many factors interacted in a circular manner to contribute to his decline. It would be utterly inadequate, for example, to conclude that the drugs were the cause of his psychosis. His use of drugs was made all the more likely by his lack of any form of social support and his membership of a gang that itself was made all the more predictable both by the lack of any stability in his life and his inability to assert himself due to his intellectual disability. The lack of support and the intellectual disability were a consequence of his mother's alcohol abuse, in turn very probably a result of the father's abusing her. The father's violent behaviour might have been due to alcohol, but it might also have been part of his unspecified psychiatric illness. As it would oversimplify matters to attribute Nemba's illness to drugs, so would it to attribute what emerged to be a schizophrenia to his father's mental disorder. It was a tangled web of potentially harmful factors, perhaps none of which alone might have caused his illness but, acting in concert, that culminated in the psychotic disarray that led him to our unit.

Isolating one or another factor is arbitrary and unhelpful. It might be more useful in terms of guiding management to divide the wide range of potentially causative events into predisposing, precipitating, perpetuating and protective risk factors.

With regard to Nemba, for example, his father's mental illness and his intellectual disability may be considered predisposing factors. The drugs and the violence associated with his gang membership were precipitating factors, and his lack of any social support and the stress of increasing contact with the police owing to his criminal activities would be likely perpetuating factors. Sadly, it is difficult to identify any protective factors in this unhappy story, and so it was difficult for us to feel in any way optimistic about his future.

I struggle to recall any psychotic episode in my clinical career that might have been solely attributable to one or another biological cause. Invariably there is a complex interplay of biological, psychological, socio-economic, cultural and other factors that interact and entangle, leading to the endpoint of a set of unique and specific symptoms, subsumed under the rather inadequate term of a schizophrenia spectrum disorder.

In this respect it is also inadequate to consider a dichotomous gene-versus-environment theory as the cause of schizophrenia. The futile debate persists; but it is crude and takes no account of current scientific knowledge, particularly in the field of genetics.

Currently, over one hundred gene variants have been associated with schizophrenia, for example, and are considered to exert relatively small, non-specific effects. It is therefore highly likely that not one gene variant but a number, acting together in various combinations, contribute to the eventual expression of schizophrenia. Furthermore, it is neither one gene nor another nor a particular environmental circumstance that leads to schizophrenia, but a complex interaction of genetic and environmental factors. For example, on exposure to cannabis a specific gene variant significantly increases the risk of developing schizophrenia. In theory, one could perform the necessary testing and, in the absence of this variant, puff away quite happily without the risk of going mad. Perhaps this being in theory should be emphasised. There is a persisting two- to threefold risk of developing schizophrenia on exposure to cannabis, and it would seem reckless – certainly with a family history of mental illness – to take this risk, regardless of one's genetic constitution.

The relatively new field of epigenetics demonstrates the inadequacies and distortions implicit in the enquiry as to whether schizophrenia, for example, is caused by one's genes or the environment. Epigenetics concerns the study of the ways in which environmental and other factors modulate genetic expression. We are not determined by our genes. An array of biological factors – including genetic factors – interact with internal and external environmental conditions in a much more fluid and dynamic way than we had perhaps previously imagined. 'Disposition' is probably a more appropriate term than 'determination'. The core element, or DNA, is composed of a fixed genetic sequence that RNA reads and translates according to need and circumstance. In another language, environmental factors modulate the way in which the genotype or genetic code is expressed as the observable phenotype.

The unease about thinking about the most intimate aspects of our inner worlds in a biological way arises from a vague and erroneous notion that something's being biological is in some way fixed and determined. It would be absurd to think that how we think and feel and act is separate from our physical selves. It is another question as to whether these physical processes can entirely account for who we are. Whether the biological basis of our consciousness, of how the feeling of who we are, is ever to be illuminated remains – for the time being and, for many, quite happily – a profound and beguiling mystery.

8

Medication and madness

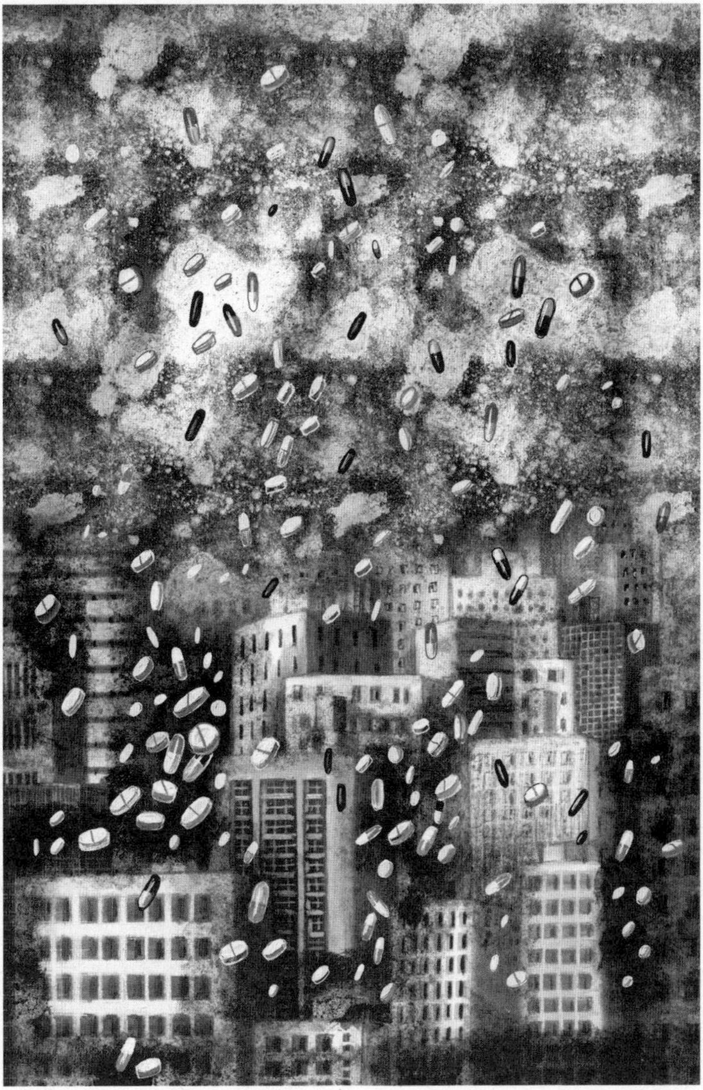

The mere idea of taking medication or using any form of physical intervention to treat mental illness is for many deeply unsettling, if not abhorrent. This is meddling with the soul. It is resorting to some crude biological instrument to change something that is infinitely complex and private. In religious terms it is challenging fate or God. It represents one of the more disturbing and wilder ambitions or expectations of modern medicine: a refusal of the acceptance of suffering, a narcissistic demand for happiness and control of the chaotic contingencies of our lives. It is the manipulation of the psyche for self-advancement or for advantage over others. It is the hubris of biomedical science, and it is without boundaries.

One contributing factor to this antagonism is the history of cruel and harmful attempts to bring madness under control. Inducing high fevers and diabetic comas, electroconvulsive therapy without anaesthesia and a wide range of psychosurgical techniques represent some of the more extreme and appalling strategies. One interpretation of this is a cruel demonstration of the power and savagery of the medical profession over the weakest and most vulnerable, and a cynical experimentation without heed of the consequences. Hope was lost; many of the patients or victims were abandoned in large asylums with no one to protect and defend them from these zealots, these mad doctors.

Another interpretation is that these interventions were attempts by the state to exert control and punish deviancy. Under the guise of medical benevolence, the capitalist order sought to maintain a compliant and homogeneous populace as a secure market for the maximisation of profit. This was dramatised in the film of the novel *One Flew Over the Cuckoo's Nest*, a fiction that to this day shapes attitudes about psychiatry and its treatments with damaging effect. That the story might represent a metaphor of how the modern state subtly exerts and maintains control over its citizens, rather than an honest and accurate account of the practice of modern psychiatry, is of little relevance. Psychiatry is perceived as sinister and its treatments as aimed to maintain social and political order rather than to benefit those suffering from mental illness.

Another way of trying to make sense of this grim past is to understand these interventions as arising from desperation. The expressions of madness were profoundly distressing and confounding and often dangerous, and the fear of madness was compounded by its origins being unknown and by the absence of effective remedies. At a time during which medicine was developing an increasingly scientific basis, psychiatry was fundamentally mysterious. It lacked a biological basis. It failed to conform to the principles of the biomedical edifice. A gastroscope could reveal a bleeding ulcer to be the cause of abdominal pain. An electrocardiogram could demonstrate the reason for somebody's suddenly putting a flat hand to his or her chest and gasping for breath. But no scope or X-ray could demonstrate the underlying cause for a psychosis, for something that was so obviously and pervasively and distressingly wrong. Nor with increasing technological sophistication could CT scans, functional MRIs, SPECT or PET scans, or any other instrument yield the neurological basis – or the biochemical or any other correlate – of mental disorders.

This is yet another cause for the disquiet and the inhibitions regarding medication and madness. It arises from an anxiety about a fundamental lack of understanding about the nature of the mind and its disorders, and about the relation of the mind to its physical substrate, the brain. These concerns arise, in turn, partly from dualist assumptions. The mind is separate from the brain. Medication can quite conceivably alter the functions of the brain, but if a fundamental dualism is accepted it is less clear, or inconceivable, how medication can affect the mind or effectively treat mental illness. The problem is not a problem if a more materialist conceptualisation of mind and brain is accepted, but these are discussions that do not take place in the turmoil of the admission unit nor in the relative calm of the outpatient clinic. For the most part, these discussions do not take place at all, but are implicit in many of the qualms that abound regarding pharmacotherapy.

The distinction between general medicine and psychiatry is not clear and nor are the methods of treatment. The precise ways in which an antihypertensive agent or a statin might exert their effects are not entirely clear – nor, certainly in primary prevention, are the benefits of these agents self-evident. Why some malignancies respond to certain cytotoxic agents and others do not is uncertain. The pharmacological treatment of a problem as common and costly as chronic pain remains controversial. There are currently no effective treatments for the dementias, or certainly no agents that significantly reverse the degenerative process. Many drugs work to a certain extent in a certain number of cases without there being a clear understanding of how and why this should be so, and this is also true of psychotropic medications.

How electroconvulsive therapy exerts its dramatic effects is unknown, but that it can be an extremely beneficial treatment in specific circumstances is not in doubt. That I have never prescribed this form of treatment has nothing to do with any misgivings about its effectiveness, despite its side-effects. Misconceptions about electroconvulsive therapy nevertheless persist, and do harm. The image of men in white coats holding down a writhing patient, usually an attractive but wild young woman, while some harridan applies the electrodes to her cruelly shaven head, continues to thrill and horrify gullible theatre and film audiences. It needs to be borne in mind that the vast majority of patients choose this form of treatment because they believe in its benefits and they are willing to tolerate the side-effects. I have not worked in any hospital anywhere where electroconvulsive therapy was administered involuntarily. I accept that this reflects only my own experience, and that the practice may be different elsewhere, but it would constitute abuse and a grave injustice.

A commonly used group of antidepressant agents, the selective serotonin reuptake inhibitors, presumably exert their benefit through an action on the serotonin neurotransmitter system. At a physiological level this is fairly immediate, and why a therapeutic response can only be expected after two to three weeks is unknown. Nor is it known with any degree of certainty how antipsychotic agents work, which complex array of inhibiting and stimulating neurotransmitters are activated, which receptor sites and secondary and tertiary messenger systems upstream and downstream are engaged, and which endophenotype changes may be required for a therapeutic response to be achieved. Not knowing how something works might be awkward or frustrating, but it has nothing to do with whether or not it works.

There are over fifty patients on the waiting list. I have to do whatever I can to make the patients currently in the ward better enough to be discharged in order to begin admitting those on the waiting list. Without effective treatments, without medication, the system would grind to a halt within weeks. We would be able neither to admit nor to discharge. When my time comes and I do not have the capacity to make informed decisions about how I should be treated, I hope I will be given whatever it takes to get me out of a situation that I have come to understand is intolerable.

A friend sent me a disturbing e-mail yesterday. A friend of hers and a patient of mine had committed suicide by jumping from a building in the city centre. The mail was of sadness and loss but was also tinged with anger and exasperation. The medication I had prescribed, she wrote, had made him normal. 'Normal' was written in capitals and followed by an exclamation mark. He had nevertheless chosen to stop the treatment. She considered his tragic and unnecessary death a consequence of this act. What madness, what other kind of madness, she wondered, had driven him to take this disastrous decision?

This is a familiar lament. 'He was doing so well, Doctor. He was back to his old self. He even said that the medication was helping him.' Then things fall apart. The vast majority of readmissions to our unit are as a result of stopping medication, often in association with substance abuse, the two of course being related. The term 'non-compliance' is discouraged in favour of 'non-adherence'. 'Non-compliance' suggests a passive acquiescence to treatment rather than an active participation in decision-making with regard to treatment options. It is surely obvious that somebody will be more willing to take the prescribed treatment if they themselves have been involved in the choice of whichever treatment might be most appropriate.

The causes of non-adherence are various and complex and interacting. It is pointless and unhelpful to blame somebody for stopping treatment, although this happens all the time. Those prescribing the treatment also bear some responsibility. It is rare that despite the clear benefits of adherence one would wilfully and for no good reason stop whatever has been prescribed. A common cause of non-adherence are side-effects; these can be severe, and from a patient's perspective outweigh the benefits of treatment. With regard to the newer 'second-generation' antipsychotic agents, weight gain, blood lipid changes, cardiac arrhythmias and somnolence are major problems. People living with severe psychiatric disorders have a life expectancy that is reduced by ten to twenty years. Many factors contribute to this shameful estimate. Those suffering from schizophrenia, for example, are very likely to smoke, not to exercise and not to take sufficient care of themselves. This in combination with the side-effects of the antipsychotic medications puts them at high risk of cardiovascular problems or heart attacks. Common side-effects of the widely used serotonin reuptake inhibitors for depression include a range of sexual problems. It seems very possible that a person would be unlikely to raise this issue with the prescribing doctor, either out of embarrassment or on the assumption that the sexual difficulty is a consequence of the depression. It is also very likely that, as a result, that person would choose to stop the treatment.

There is also a rather bizarre assumption among many doctors that it is ill-advised to inform patients of the side-effects that can be expected on taking medication. This is confused. It is not as if by not informing of side-effects they are less likely to occur. The reasoning seems to be that the patient will be deterred from taking the medication. On the contrary, somebody is much more likely to adhere to the prescribed treatment if they are informed of the reason why the medication is being prescribed and which side-effects they can expect. They might, then, hopefully be in a better position to make an informed decision, weighing possible benefits against the predictable side-effects, and therefore much more likely to adhere. Not providing adequate information is patronising and unhelpful.

Such information is not limited to possible side-effects but should also include, among many items, the indications for the treatment in the first place, a possible delayed onset of action and the necessary duration of treatment. It is difficult to imagine why one should be expected to begin whichever treatment is prescribed without knowing why. The antidepressant effects of the selective serotonin reuptake inhibitors can only be anticipated after two to four weeks. It is to be expected that, not being informed of this delayed onset of action, a depressed and angry patient will throw the tablets down the lavatory. It can also be anticipated that somebody would be very likely to stop the treatment once he or she felt better, certainly if side-effects were experienced. It is not at all self-evident that one should continue the prescribed psychotropic for six to twelve months, as one should, even though there has been a positive response. Blaming a patient for non-adherence in such circumstances is ridiculous. These difficulties are of course not confined to psychiatry – any doctor prescribing treatment for usually chronic conditions, commonly tuberculosis or HIV in South Africa, will be familiar with these problems that are not insurmountable, however confounding they might at times seem.

There are many other prosaic, but important, reasons why somebody might not continue a form of treatment that confers a benefit – or at least reduces significantly the likelihood of readmission to hospital. The cost of transport to the clinic, the habit of gangsters of congregating near the clinic to prey on those collecting disability grants, and the stigma associated with attendance at a separate psychiatric clinic are common explanations given by both patients and families. There are other perhaps more subtle and difficult factors that are less remediable. On each occasion that a medication is administered, an onerous and possibly contradictory message is given – that one is mad, that without the treatment one would be in hospital, that deep down one is sick and it is only this extraneous, banal pharmacological thing that controls or suppresses this miserable truth. In this context, a lack of enthusiastic adherence is understandable. There is no escape.

There is another factor contributing not necessarily to a refusal of treatment but to a reluctance or ambivalence. Psychotic symptoms in the form of delusions and hallucinations may be conceptualised as secondary phenomena, or attempts to give meaningful form to biological or neurological events that are experienced as intolerable and menacing. Psychotic phenomena may represent a struggle to recover control and, however incomprehensible it might seem from the outside, restore meaning and coherence in a terrifying and formless world. The phasic nature of symptoms is perhaps not sufficiently registered. Psychotic symptoms come and go. Patients say, 'Somebody is trying to kill me. I know you think I'm mad but it's true,' and then, 'I felt as if somebody was trying to kill me,' and then, 'I was crazy – it's gone.' It does not seem inconceivable that, at least in some instances, symptoms represent strategies for levering oneself out of the abyss.

For as long as I have known him, Manuel has been cheerful and enthusiastic. When I see him in the outpatient clinic he greets me warmly. He is dishevelled. His hair is long and unkempt and his clothes are dirty. Although it is summer he is wearing a thick jersey. He is a graduate of the university I attended. He won the class medal in the physics department and was embarking on a doctorate before this wretched illness turned his life upside down. He appears unfazed. He tells me he is delighted with his medication. It is 'perfect', he says in wonder. He sternly insists that I am under no circumstances allowed to alter it. He is floridly psychotic. The reasons for his apparent excitement and his expressed gratitude for this supposedly successful treatment are mysterious to me. I have not taken the symptoms away. He has not recovered, yet he appears to be content. This, it seems, is what he wants. His ailment has been acknowledged. He is receiving treatment. This appears to be more important to him than any benefit he might gain.

This calls into question the goals of treatment – or more specifically antipsychotic medication. In my practice I wanted to change the term to 'neuro-modulation', which might be rather abstruse. My ambitions met with no success. If symptoms do represent tentative steps to recovery, the elimination of these symptoms would not necessarily be helpful and would instead leave a void. The distress and disability associated with psychotic symptoms are the more appropriate focus of therapeutic attention. Acknowledging and affirming a person's vivid experience and the struggle towards recovery – and simultaneously seeking to modulate or attenuate the intense distress and confusion that is part of the process – requires a difficult and at times elusive balance.

9

Traditional healers, Freud, Jung and other interpreters

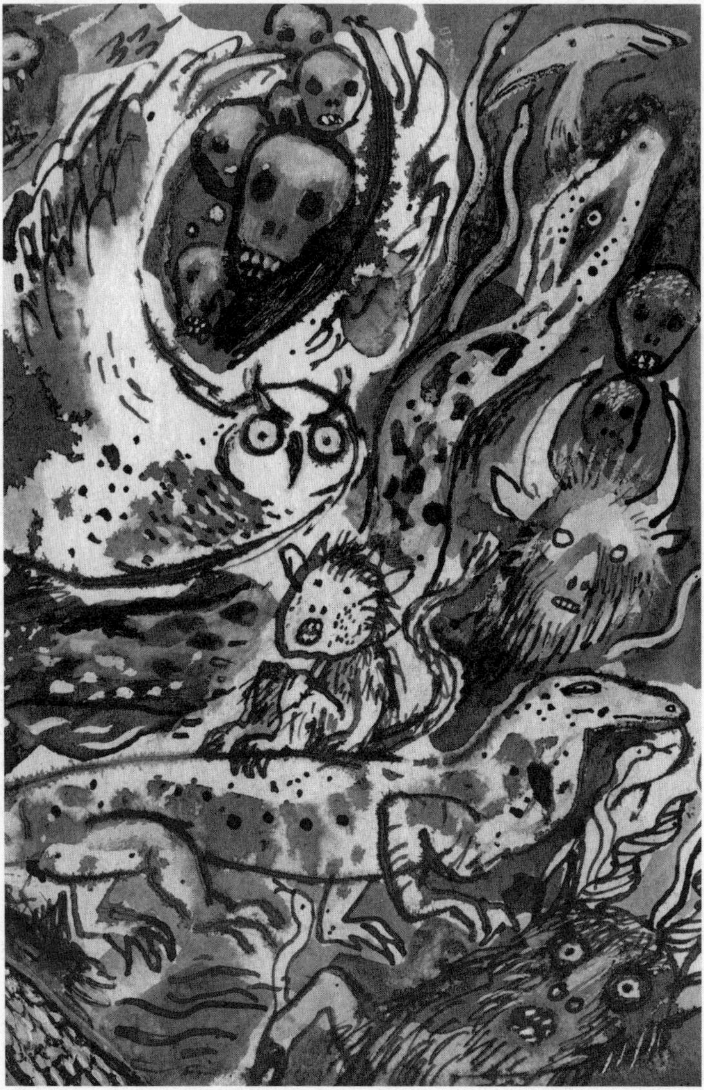

'She comes to fetch me … she comes to fetch my heart … she comes to fetch my breathing …'

Michel is a twenty-one-year-old, single, unemployed man originally from Burundi. He made his way slowly through Tanzania to Mozambique, and thence to KwaZulu-Natal and finally to the Western Cape. He was initially accompanied by his father but when they reached the relative safety of Tanzania the father had returned to Burundi to collect his wife and a younger son. The father and son were killed in Burundi; the mother disappeared and was presumed also to have been killed.

As Michel moved southwards, without family or any other form of support, he gradually developed the belief that his body and his life had been overtaken by a woman he named Maji Kali. In desperation, while in KwaZulu-Natal he had sought help from a traditional healer. He had been advised to perform certain rituals and was given a red rope to tie around his waist. This was to no avail. Having moved to Cape Town, he tried to hang himself because he found the presence of this woman intolerable. He was admitted to hospital where he again requested the help of a sangoma. He said, 'You can't do magic, I can't do magic … only magic can help me …'

He says that he is not angry or afraid, but acknowledges that he is profoundly depressed. A large part of the depression is his helplessness. He is in the wrong place. There is no possibility that we can help him by keeping him in the hospital. The only solution appears to be magical, and that can only be provided by a traditional healer. It seems that the desperate nature of his situation calls for the certainty of magic, however impossible that might be. He seeks a cure for his intractable problems. He is not interested in how this belief might have arisen, or how Maji Kali might have emerged in his world. He holds Maji Kali to account for his predicament. He needs a remedy that will guarantee her expulsion from his world. An interpretation has been made and now it is for the sangoma to do whatever is necessary to undo the tragedies of his life, to do the magic, to make things whole again. We are keeping him in hospital against his will.

On a psychological level, clearly Michel feels that he has lost control over the circumstances of his life. This control has been granted to Maji Kali who provides in some sort of concrete way an explanation for the losses he has suffered. How to manage this poses a certain difficulty in that the delusion provides him with a meaningful account of what has happened to him. With successful treatment – the elimination of Maji Kali – what should then be made of his predicament? We would be taking away a hope of restoration, however illusory.

Michel is treated with conventional antipsychotic medication and arrangements are made to bring a traditional healer to the hospital to advise on traditionally meaningful ways of dealing with Maji Kali. After approximately two weeks Michel is discharged from the hospital to a refugee centre. Maji Kali has disappeared. The extent to which the belief in her and the rituals of her expulsion contributed to his recovery is unclear. What is more sadly clear to us in this context are the limitations of what might constitute recovery. He is a young man in a foreign country with no family and no support and no better prospect of a future than the one he had before he came to our hospital. The sangoma is not able to undo his terrible misfortunes. Nor are we.

Mandla is a law student at the university to which the hospital is affiliated. He is in the third year of his course and is flourishing academically. He is the pride and hope of his family, who live in the Eastern Cape. His colleagues and teachers have become increasingly concerned about his erratic and uncharacteristic behaviour. Their alarm increases when he stops attending lectures. He is admitted to our unit in an overtly psychotic state. He is not in any way distressed, but rather elated or illuminated. He has received the calling to be a traditional healer, he tells us. This is *ukuthwasa*, and it cannot be resisted. Refusal to answer the calling will cause displeasure to the ancestors and result in prolonged personal suffering. There is no choice other than to abandon his career as a lawyer and embark on his training to become a healer.

This causes consternation and dismay among his family. Informed by the university of his admission to our hospital, they immediately make their long way from the rural Eastern Cape to the city. They dismiss his claim of having been called. That is the past. That is traditionalist, and has no part in the future they envision for him as a bright young professional in a western world. He cannot be allowed to drag them backwards after all the sacrifices that have been made to get him as far as he has come. They are angry and anxious and plead with us to ignore his talk of *ukuthwasa* and to treat him conventionally so that he can be discharged as soon as possible to resume his studies.

In accordance with the family's wishes, and as he does not refuse treatment, conventional antipsychotic medications are prescribed and the symptoms resolve. At the time of his discharge Mandla seems mystified by what happened. He does not want to become a healer. He is determined to become a lawyer, a source of pride to his family and community. He is to be part of the vanguard of the new South Africa.

He is readmitted within six months. He is not so sure, now, about what might be happening to him, and nor is his family. Perhaps this *ukuthwasa* is true, although they do not want it to be. Perhaps it is just too powerful to be refused. Perhaps they will have to put aside their dreams of a different future. Another course of antipsychotic medication is not going to resolve these issues.

Enquiries are made and we manage to find a healer who is prepared to come to the hospital and meet with us to decide how we should proceed. We are a little disappointed when he arrives. Perhaps we are hoping for something more exotic, for him to be half-naked and covered in animal skins and wearing some sort of headdress with feathers to terrify and cast down the evil spirits. Mr Malosi is dressed in a suit and tie with only a simple string of beads and a staff to signify his calling. He is pleasant and mild-mannered but curiously insistent that I should address him as 'professor' while he calls me 'darling'. It is not to be a conventional clinical meeting. Everybody involved is in attendance: Mandla and his family, Mr or Professor Malosi, our clinical team of doctors, psychologists, social workers and occupational therapists, and a number of bemused nurses and students. I say that I do not think that Mandla is going to be able to manage without the medication. Mr Malosi proposes a collaboration. We should continue with our treatment and inform him when we plan to discharge Mandla. On Mandla's discharge, Mr Malosi insists that he will ensure that Mandla continues his medication while at the same time undergoing the rituals for becoming a healer. He does not think that being a traditional healer is incompatible with being a lawyer. He advises that Mandla continue with his studies and again he promises to provide support and supervise. I think we are all relieved and also reassured by this flexible and imaginative course of action. We all fervently hope it will work when we wish him well on his discharge a week later.

This encounter raises the hope of a more constructive relationship between ourselves and the traditional healers, whom many of our patients have consulted before they get to us. Given the far greater numbers of healers in the communities of southern Africa, and a shared culture and a meaningful idiom of misfortune and disease, there seems to be an important opportunity to work together, a possibility of integrating understanding and explanation in the provision of a more effective service to our patients. Another encounter cautioned us against any naïve assumptions, although I continue to believe that finding imaginative ways of collaborating between traditional healers and western, evidence-based approaches is necessary and important and a possibly innovative and creative way of dealing with otherwise intractable problems.

Zwelethu was discharged from our unit six months ago. The diagnosis was made of a schizophrenic illness and he responded well to the prescribed antipsychotic medication. The details of what happened subsequently are not clear. He returned to his family in a rural area of the province. It seems very possible that he stopped his medication at some stage. He became ill and his family took him to consult a group of traditional healers. The diagnosis on this occasion was possession by an evil spirit. The remedy was to place stones over an open fire, and then to throw water on the stones with the expectation that the scalding heat would drive out the evil spirits. When Zwelethu struggled against the terrible pain of his burning skin this was interpreted as evidence of the evil spirit fighting against the treatment and he was held down over the stones with greater force.

On his return to our unit Zwelethu has been mutilated. He has lost most of his nose to burn injuries, he is blind in one eye and he is missing fingers on both his left and right hands. Whatever evil spirits there might have been are dismissed within a few days of antipsychotic medication. His family are grief-stricken and enraged.

One of the many issues raised in this story is the problem of interpretation. Seeking evidence is not the sole province of a western-oriented, scientific approach to medicine. In this account of what happened to Zwelethu, psychotic symptoms were interpreted as evidence of being possessed by evil spirits. In a further cruel elaboration, his understandable struggle to escape was interpreted as further evidence of possession. The unbearable suffering inflicted by the treatment was then rationalised as a necessarily extreme measure to heal this most unfortunate man. In some grotesque way, and most likely to the perpetrators of this abuse, it might have all made sense and been justified.

It is perhaps needlessly provocative and ridiculous to associate Freud and Jung and others with these practices. The argument is against interpretation. It concerns the possible harm done in not attending to what is presented, but rather in interpreting the problem that presents itself in terms of something else. That something else might be the belief in evil spirits or some other less malign school of thought or doctrine or ideology.

In my training to become a doctor and then a specialist psychiatrist, psychoanalysis had very little influence. I am therefore in no position to make any critical comment about the theory and practice of the various schools of psychoanalysis, other than to recount my own troubled experience. For a few months I was required to attend a specialist and renowned psychoanalytic unit in London. It was at the time of great concern about the sexual abuse of children and how this should be managed. As students we watched through a one-way mirror as a family was interviewed. It was suspected that the father had abused his daughter. Much is made in modern medicine and psychiatry about the need for evidence, but again this raises the question of what constitutes evidence. In this miserable circumstance it seemed that the father's silence or his failure to divulge was considered evidence of his complicity. The long, awkward pauses, the confusion and the excruciating tensions were interpreted, or at least it seemed to me, as repression and denial. The family was trapped. The truth would be revealed and, if not, that was indicative of the power of defensive strategies. In all my years of training I struggle to recall a time when I have felt more ill at ease, as if I should not have been there.

At the same institution my senior colleagues talked enthusiastically of the 'material' that was brought to therapy sessions. This again caused us disquiet, as if the deeply personal and complex stories of distress and pain were being used to confirm and bolster an abstract edifice that could not have made any sense to those bewildered participants in the therapy sessions. To have your private anguish interpreted by a remote and dispassionate therapist as a repressed desire to have sex with your mother and kill your father, or as any other myth, seems more likely to offend and alienate than be helpful. It also seemed to us at the time to be absurd.

The causes of schizophrenia and of autism remain unknown. In the psychoanalytical culture of the middle of the twentieth century, this did not deter proponents from declaring that the causes – if not the blame – for these immensely complex disorders lay with the mothers. Without any evidence, but in accordance with psychoanalytic doctrine, the cold, disengaged mother was held to account. This heedlessly and unnecessarily compounded the distress of affected families.

Jung and others within the psychoanalytic tradition have had little impact on standard psychiatric thinking and practice at the beginning of the twenty-first century, certainly with regard to serious mental illnesses, given the problems that that terminology entails. More specifically, the interpretation of dreams in regard to schizophrenia is irrelevant, although Jung did not seem to hesitate to make a diagnosis of schizophrenia on the basis of his interpretation of dreams. This seemed to take precedence over a patient's personal history and social context. The interpretations, anyway, very often seem idiosyncratic – if not bizarre – and had more to do with Jung's spiritual, mystical and neo-pagan preoccupations than with his patients' predicaments. I should admit to being discouraged by his own account of what he seemed to regard as a 'blissful' revelation involving God defecating on a cathedral with such explosive force that it was destroyed. The young Carl Jung describes weeping with joy and gratitude at his interpretation of this lurid image as an indication that 'one should be utterly abandoned to God'. On rereading this account in *Memories, Dreams, Reflections* it is opaque to me as to how he came to draw this enraptured conclusion from the divine detonation.

The issue is less with the details of these various and fragmented and at times mutually hostile explanatory models. The concern is with an inappropriate foreclosure, an explaining away, whether that might be as evil spirits or an oedipal complex or some arcane governing archetype of a collective unconscious. This does not indicate a presumptuous rejection of these schools of thinking, and it is possible that the experiences described merely reflect a crude and reductionist application of sophisticated psychoanalytical principles, and that these ways of thinking might have greater meaning in other domains of psychiatry. It does suggest that, with regard to the understanding and treatment of schizophrenia and other serious psychiatric disorders, psychoanalysis has a minimal and waning relevance.

10

Coercion

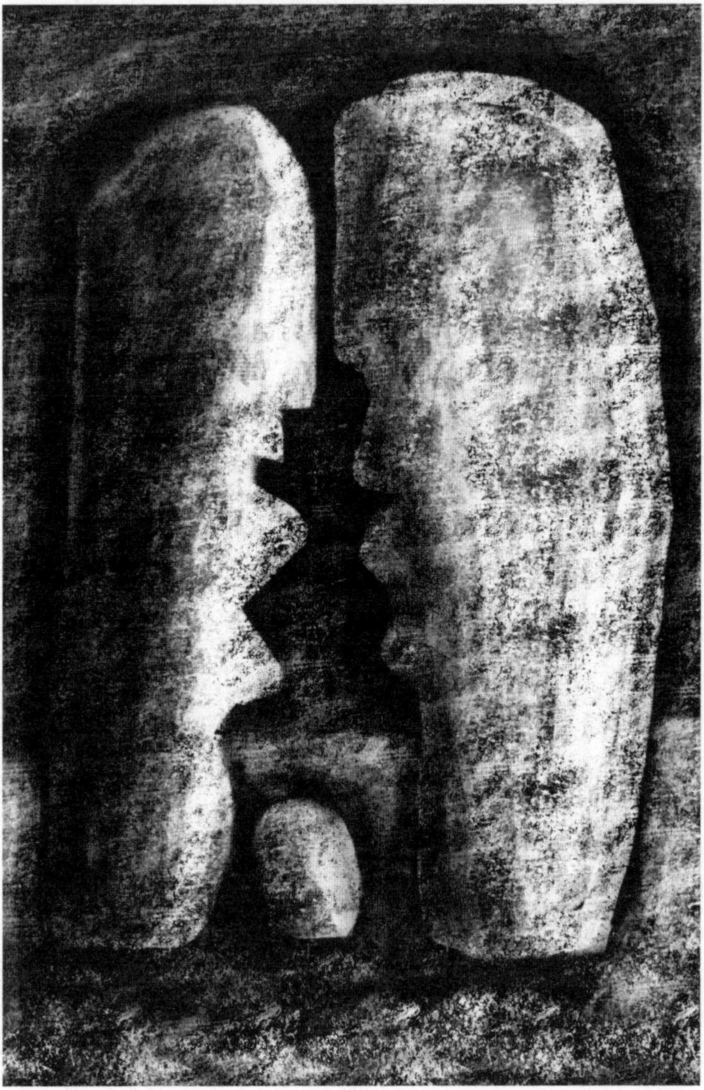

This is a fiction that might be familiar to many of us, in various permutations.

Someone has gone crazy. He has run amok. He is charging around, shouting and screaming. He is not dangerous but he is disturbing the peace. He is rattling the order of things. Perhaps he is embarrassing. Perhaps, at another level, his behaviour is disconcerting. He is defying the unwritten rules of how we should be together. In this respect he is threatening. He does not belong. Perhaps he is mad in that it is madness not to conform, to know how to behave in order to serve one's own needs and the needs of society. He is out of control and that cannot be allowed. Anything could happen. Who knows how it will end? Something must be done. He needs to be removed.

The police are summoned. There is no evidence of criminal behaviour, so an ambulance is called. It does not matter too much how he is removed, as long as peace and order are restored. Men in long white coats bundle him into the back of the ambulance; perhaps a siren is sounded as he is rushed away to some dark and foreboding asylum beyond the outskirts of the city. There he is injected with powerful sedating substances. He is not assessed in any way. There are no formal admitting procedures. He is put into a uniform and dragged semi-comatose into a single room that looks like a prison cell. When he regains consciousness, he is frightened and angry. He protests loudly and three burly and menacing male nurses restrain him and sedate him again.

When he recovers again, he decides to adopt a different strategy. He tries to reason with the nurses. He says he is well now, that he does not belong in hospital. Something happened that he does not fully understand but it is over and he needs to go. This to the staff is a clear indication that he has no insight and that he should remain in hospital and receive further medication. The patient becomes increasingly distressed. He demands to see a doctor.

Eventually a psychiatrist is summoned. This is a sinister, rather dishevelled, middle-aged man in a grubby long white coat. Perhaps he sneers. Perhaps he has a tremor. He is drunk. No, better, he is a drunken psychopath! The doctor is wrestling with his own demons! He does not ask any questions but he peers at the patient as if he is a specimen. He confers with the nurses. Not understanding the need for further treatment, the patient is deemed uncooperative and more medication is prescribed. Perhaps the race angle needs to be addressed: the doctor is white and the patient is black. Violence is perpetrated on the black body. There is no good reason to stop at race. The doctor is privileged, middle-class, a beneficiary of an unequal socioeconomic and educational system. The patient is disempowered. The violence of structural and historical injustices is enacted and perpetuated.

The patient perceives his situation as hopeless. He has no voice, or his voice is disallowed. He becomes apathetic. He refuses to eat and drink in some confused way as an act of self-assertion. This is interpreted as indicating a depressive disorder. Electroconvulsive therapy is prescribed. No permission is sought as he is considered to lack the capacity for informed consent. This could go on and on. Maybe it could be taken to a further extreme. A lobotomy is proposed, either due to his perceived failure to respond to treatment or as punishment for his intransigence.

This ludicrous scenario may be regarded as a harmless fiction. It is not. It is odious and deeply offensive and it causes harm. Our ways of thinking are shaped insidiously by such melodramatic and sensational depictions. Reality is too grim, or too prosaic, or too boring.

I am not sure to what extent this lurid depiction of cruel and coercive activity informs thinking about current psychiatric practice. It certainly reflects, to a greater or lesser extent, portrayals in popular film and theatre. The problem then arises that it is too easy to dismiss these absurd melodramas as mere fiction, or the shrill and hostile distortions of one or another anti-psychiatry or propagandist position. Insufficient heed is then paid to the very real and complex problems of relations of power, and the associated quandaries of coercion in the practice of psychiatry, however well-intended and formalised in law these practices might be.

An alternative scenario might be described, based on a composite of a number of clinical encounters in which I have been involved.

Nxaba has begun to act strangely over the past few days. He has become withdrawn and hostile towards his friends and family. He starts to mutter to himself and refuses or is unable to say what might be troubling him. The family of six live in a two-roomed shack in an informal settlement. The mother begins to worry about the safety of the younger siblings who share a room with Nxaba. A crisis develops in the early hours of the morning when the mother wakes to the smell of burning and the terrifying crackle of flames. Nxaba has set fire to his bed and locked the door of the room, trapping his younger siblings. With the help of neighbours the father manages to break down the door and rescue the children. They also manage to douse the flames and prevent a conflagration engulfing the adjacent dwellings.

Nxaba is unable to explain his actions. He appears to be confused. He tells his father in a disjointed jumble of words that he felt compelled to burn down the house, that the voices were telling him that this is what he had to do. He shows no sign of remorse and no awareness of the grave dangerousness of his actions. The father stays with his son in one of the rooms for the night. Nobody can sleep. Everybody is afraid.

The next morning the father tells Nxaba he is taking him to the local clinic. He says he thinks the son is sick and that the situation is dangerous. The whole neighbourhood could have gone up in flames. Nxaba refuses to accompany his father. He says there is nothing wrong with him. With the help of the angry and frightened neighbours, Nxaba is forced into a taxi and taken to the clinic. There he is assessed by a nursing sister and examined by a doctor. There appears to be no evidence of a medical condition to account for his strange behaviour. A number of investigations are performed and exclude any likelihood that drugs might have been the cause. Nxaba continues to behave in a hostile and disorganised way. He insists that he has to leave the clinic; in a menacing way, he says that he has unfinished business. Although he does not say anything explicit about them, it becomes clear to the clinic staff that he is responding to voices over which he appears to have no control.

The staff form the opinion that he is probably suffering from some form of mental illness, that he is refusing or unable to accept that he is ill and needs treatment and that, as a consequence, he poses a danger to himself and to others. The father signs an application form and the nursing sister and the doctor sign the necessary forms for involuntary care. Nxaba continues to insist that he must go. For his own safety and the safety of others, a decision is made that he should be kept in a closed ward. He is assessed again the following day and the day after by two medical practitioners who agree that he is ill and needs treatment. After three days there is no sign of improvement so the legal forms are completed for Nxaba to be transferred to a specialist unit. These forms are sent to an independent review board whose task it is to ensure that the rights of a patients in predicaments such as Nxaba's are respected. The forms are also sent to a judge in chambers to ensure that the process is in accordance with the letter and spirit of the Mental Health Care Act.

However well-intended to protect against the possible abuses described in the first scenario, these processes are fraught with complications. One right may conflict with another. One ethical principle may be inconsistent with another. Nxaba has a right to receive treatment. He also has the right to refuse treatment. The principle of beneficence requires that he be treated for what quite obviously is a serious illness that is causing him and his family great distress. This conflicts with the principle of autonomy, in this circumstance the need to respect his refusal of treatment. The difficulties arise to some extent from the problematic notion of insight. An argument could be made that, due to his impaired insight, the right to refuse treatment is ceded, and for the same reason beneficence should take precedence over autonomy. This might be dismissed as being paternalistic.

Another difficulty is that insight is a rather abstract concept. There are degrees of insight, and these might shift over time. Nxaba, for example, might have some insight that he is unwell but no insight into the need for treatment. Differences in cultural attitudes can compound these difficulties. Nxaba may accept that he is ill but attribute this to bewitchment. On these grounds he might insist that he be seen by a traditional healer rather than treated in a western-oriented, evidence-based context that he perceives to be alien. In this regard it seems very likely that he would regard decisions made about his care according to the principle of beneficence as being coercive.

These cultural differences arise not infrequently and need to be addressed with great care. It is not at all helpful to have one's belief in, for example, *amafufunyana* dismissed as having no scientific foundation. Regardless of the science, the belief does provide some form of an explanation. It grants meaning. An explanation of synaptic dysconnectivity in the central nervous system is not going to be meaningful to Nxaba and his family, nor does any kind of scientific explanation answer the urgent question as to why the problem might have arisen in the first place. Disregard of the cultural context, and the meanings and explanations that families and patients attach to the symptoms of mental illness, can constitute another, less concrete form of coercion.

A scientific evidence-based approach does not need to be antagonistic to a more traditionalist, culture-specific position. There is no good reason to believe it is one thing or another, and a more creative complementariness needs to be adopted. Understanding and explanation should not be considered to be in binary opposition; there might be many levels of explanation, some more speculative, others based on sound evidence.

Some degree of coercion might be inevitable in the management of extreme psychotic states, given that a defining feature of the psychoses is a lack of insight. That lack of insight might be into the dangerousness of psychotic phenomena such as command hallucinations or persecutory delusions. This can, of course, only be ethically justifiable on the basis of an assumption that the treatment given involuntarily can reasonably be expected to be effective in relieving the symptoms and hence reducing the risk of dangerousness.

Maluti says, 'I don't want to die but the voices are telling me to kill myself. If I don't obey my whole family will be killed. My village will be burned to the ground. There is absolutely nothing I can do about it. You cannot and you must not stop me. You do not understand. I am not ill. I do not need any treatment. I just need to do what the voices are telling me to do. Leave me alone. I have to die. The voices are telling me this.'

Qama has savagely attacked his mother and nearly killed her. He insists that she is not his mother but an evil spirit who has taken the form of his mother and bewitched him, that he had to destroy this evil spirit to protect both himself and his mother.

Wishing to avoid coercion, I have made errors of clinical judgement that have had tragic consequences. A young student was admitted to our unit following a suicide attempt. After about five days in the high care unit he pleaded with us to be allowed out for a day. He did not ask to be discharged. He said that he was feeling restless and confined. The noise on the ward was distressing him and he was having difficulty in regaining the strength of mind and the determination necessary to resolve the problems that had led to what seemed a precipitous attempt to end his life. He was not psychotic. He spoke with insight and reasonably. His concerns were understandable. A turbulent admission unit accommodating for the most part behaviourally disturbed, psychotic young men, many from very different backgrounds from his and possibly perceived by this young student to be threatening, was clearly not an environment conducive to his recovery.

'You have to let me out for a few hours. I promise you I will come back. I won't be on my own. I've got friends who will look after me. I don't know why I did that. It was something impulsive and I do not feel that way now. I don't want to end my life. I want to live. But being here is not helping me. Please. You cannot understand what it is like being locked up here. How can I possibly get better? It is safer for me to be out of here. I am not going to do anything silly. I will be all right. Please. Let me go, just for the night. I will come back. I promise. I know I need help. I want to get better. You must trust me. Please.'

His friends confirmed that they would look after him. They would be vigilant. They would take turns to watch over him and they would return him to the unit the following afternoon. If all went well, I made an assurance on my own part that we would plan to discharge him within the week.

Early the next morning I was informed that he had been found hanging in the bedroom of the friends' home.

To this day, I am not sure that in retrospect I would have made a different decision. It was nevertheless a terribly bad decision, and I regretted it profoundly. I needed to show trust in him. I wanted to act in good faith. I wanted there to be hope but I was wrong and a bright healthy young man died. It could and should have been prevented and it was not possible for me to think that I was not responsible.

Acting under pressure from colleagues, from families, from managers and, in this last awful incident, from patients themselves escalates the likelihood of things going wrong, but I struggle to imagine how things might be otherwise. There is no escaping risk. There is no escaping uncertainty and there are no guarantees that the decision made is the right decision.

In these deeply distressing circumstances it is difficult for me to imagine how a degree of coercion might not be avoidable, as a temporary measure, with the intention of acting in the best interest of our patients, and given their lack of capacity owing to illness.

It is nevertheless one of the most difficult things I have had to cope with in clinical practice.

11

Violence

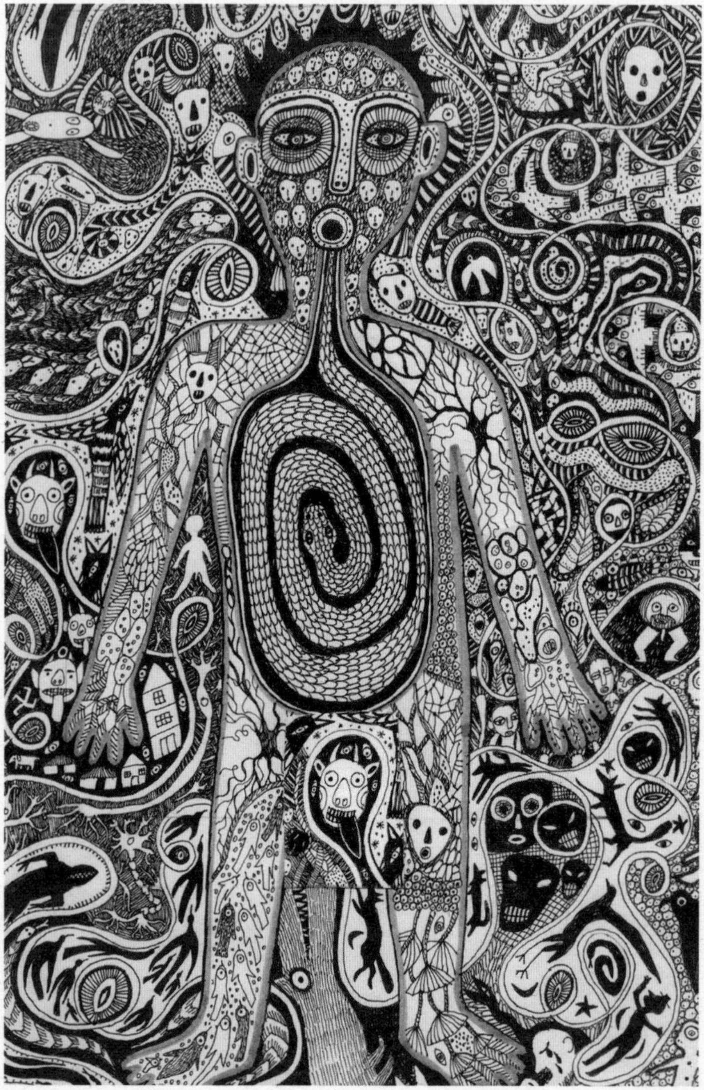

'I am an assassin.'

'An assassin?'

'Yes. I am the assassin.'

'Who do you plan to assassinate?'

'The president. Of course.'

'Oh, the president. Of which country?'

'This country. Of course.'

'When do you plan to undertake this assassination?'

'When the time is ready.'

'Why do you want to assassinate the president?'

'I don't want to assassinate him. It is just something that I have to do.'

'What do you mean, it is just something you have to do?'

'There are forces, very powerful forces or spirits, that are compelling me to do this. It is outside my control.'

'Don't you think it is wrong – to kill anybody, whether or not it is the president?'

Unathi is vague. 'Yes, I think it is probably wrong, but it is not up to me. It is not for me to decide whether or not it is the right or wrong thing to do. It will just happen. When the time comes.'

'How do you know when that will be?'

'When the forces of energy reach my penis.'

'What do you mean?'

'The forces are moving slowly through my body. I can feel them moving from my head into my chest. They are moving very slowly. When they get into my penis I will know the time has come.'

'How will you know that the forces have reached your penis?'

'When it gets long.'

'How long?'

'Nine inches.'

'When your penis reaches nine inches in length you will know it is time to kill the president of the country?'

'Yes. That is right.'

He speaks without emotion, but patiently, as if explaining something that is self-evident, as if I should know these things. He is untroubled.

'You do understand I have responsibilities?'

'What do you mean, responsibilities?'

'If I have reason to believe that the life of the president of the country, or anybody else for that matter, is in danger, I have a duty to inform that person.'

'No. That is ridiculous.'

'What do you mean, it is ridiculous?'

'His life is not in danger.'

'Why not?'

'Because my penis is not long enough.'

'And when it is?'

Unathi hesitates. 'Then I will be the assassin.'

'How will I know that your penis has become long enough for you to be an assassin?'

'I will tell you.'

'You will come and tell me when your penis is nine inches long so that I can inform the president that his life is in danger? How can I rely on you? You understand that I must inform the security services of this plan to assassinate the president. There is a risk.'

'Yes.' He seems nonchalant.

'And what if you are then arrested, and charged with a very grave offence?'

He shrugs. This appears to be of no concern to him. 'I don't know. Things will just happen. I can't stop anything. It is not for me to decide what to do.'

I am in a dilemma. I do not doubt that Unathi will act when the time comes. I do not doubt that he poses a danger, but the danger is not imminent.

It is also difficult for me to imagine contacting the president's security office to inform them that my patient intends to murder him when his penis has reached a length of nine inches. It seems quite possible that they will become suspicious of me. Do I think this is amusing? Am I trying to make a joke of the threatened assassination of the president? Are psychiatrists all mad?

I make an appointment to see Unathi in a month's time. On this occasion, he is quite cheerful. He seems to want to reassure me. The forces are still in his chest. They have barely moved. They are nowhere near his penis. I must not worry. There is no immediate danger to the president.

'I am fine. You must not worry. Everything is okay,' he tells me. He is not yet an assassin.

We wait.

The association of violence with mental illness is a significant contributing factor to the burden of stigma. The crazed killer is a familiar figure in the popular imagination, fuelled by fictional accounts in film, theatre and other media that feed on our apparent need to be titillated by violence. Psychopathy is characterised as psychosis. He was attacked in a psychotic frenzy. A psychopathic killer is on the loose. He, and invariably it is a he, has to be a psychopath because of the evil brutality of his actions. The terminology of mental illness is used without seriously implying that these acts were committed owing to mental illness. It is merely a matter of degree. The acts were beyond the pale, inhuman. This evil could not possibly have been committed by a sane person, by one of us. Madness is carelessly invoked.

Mental-health-care workers, a term used to indicate the very wide range of professionals engaged in the field, strive to correct this misapprehension. Most of us consider it our duty to do everything we possibly can to reduce the alienating and harmful effects of stigma. To this end we make the claim repeatedly that people with mental illnesses are no more violent than those without a diagnosis of mental illness. This applies particularly to the spectrum of serious mental illnesses or psychoses, accepting the problematic nature of this terminology. It is not in any way suggested that anxiety and depression are not serious mental-health problems, but these conditions are not associated with violence.

The claim of a lack of association of psychosis with violence needs to be qualified. With adequate social support, a person living with schizophrenia who does not use recreational drugs and who is adherent to treatment is no more likely to be violent than a member of the general population. This does not apply to a young man with a long history of a severe psychotic illness with frequent relapses owing to non-adherence to treatment and substance-abuse problems and no social support. The risk of dangerousness increases when such a person is responding to command hallucinations, telling him or her to do things over which he or she feels he or she has no control.

'Kill her, she is a witch!'

'You are a worthless person. You do not deserve to be alive. Why don't you just end it? Do it! Now!'

In this respect Unathi has to be considered potentially dangerous. He feels he has no agency. He has been compelled by external forces to become an assassin. There is no assumption of a freedom of choice, of ourselves as autonomous or of the will being free. He is fated to be the assassin.

Yet I do not believe that Unathi in his present state poses a danger to the president of the country. This is a clinical judgement and I might be gravely wrong, in which case there will be severe repercussions with regard not just to the life of the president but also to my career. There are a number of reasons to consider this not to be a matter of urgency, one being the banal observation that the president is inclined to surround himself with a phalanx of bodyguards, and to travel around the country in a cavalcade of security vehicles with flashing blue lights and menacing outriders. Another reason is the very nature of his psychotic illness.

Although he is extremely intelligent Unathi's resources for planning and problem-solving have become severely impaired, associated with his diminished insight and judgement. It is highly improbable that Unathi has the capacity for the very complicated processes that would be required to take out the president successfully. A more likely scenario would be that when the time came he would make his way to the Houses of Parliament. When asked by the security staff what his business was, he might say politely – and with due deference to authority – that he has come to assassinate the president. He might even be asked why he would want to do such a terrible thing. When he answers that his penis is now long enough things would take a predictable course. This seems more probable but it is not certain. Violence is unpredictable.

It is also complex. A wide range of differentially weighted factors contribute to the emergence of violence. Because somebody has a diagnosis of a mental illness it cannot be assumed that if he or she commits an act of violence it should be attributed to the mental illness. More specifically, if a person suffers from schizophrenia or any other psychotic illness there is no reason to believe that an act of violence that he or she commits may be directly due to the psychosis. Other problems, most obviously substance abuse, may provide a more plausible explanation. Probably more common are social and economic factors. A person with a diagnosis of schizophrenia is very likely to experience exclusion and as a result of the illness and the incapacity to work to drift down the social scale. A predictable recourse to drug use and the absence of any meaningful social support will put that person at high risk of violence, either as a victim or as a perpetrator. In this scenario mental illness is certainly a contributory factor – but the absence of social cohesion as a protective influence and the substance abuse as a precipitating element might have a more significant bearing on the violence committed.

Command hallucinations – a voice or voices experienced in external space instructing somebody to do something, usually in the context of schizophrenia – pose a particular threat of violence. This again needs qualification. There are degrees of agency. A person might hear a voice telling him to kill his mother but have a sufficient sense of self or autonomy to refuse this action. He might have a degree of insight leading him to recognise the commanding voice as a symptom of his illness. He might on the other hand believe he has no power at all to resist the voices, commit an act of violence and thereafter deny any responsibility, insisting, 'It was the voices that made me do it. I had no control. How could I do such a terrible thing? It was not me.'

It is the early afternoon of 6 September 1966 in the House of Assembly in Cape Town. Prime Minister Hendrik Verwoerd has just entered the House for the afternoon session. He makes his way to the front bench and exchanges greetings with his parliamentary colleagues. Just as he takes his seat a uniformed parliamentary messenger bustles across the floor from the lobby entrance. The name of this messenger is Dmitri Tsafendas. Without warning Tsafendas draws a sheathed knife from his clothing. He bends over the prime minister and withdraws the knife from the sheath. He stabs Dr Verwoerd in the neck and chest four times. Members of Parliament rush forward to subdue him. Others, among them four medical doctors, go to the aid of the prime minister. Frantic attempts at resuscitation are made. Dr Verwoerd is rushed to Groote Schuur Hospital where he is pronounced dead on arrival.

Dmitri Tsafendas was born in Lourenço Marques to a Greek seaman and a Mozambican woman of mixed race. He was sent to live with a grandmother in Egypt in the first year of his life. He returned to Mozambique five years later and at the age of ten he moved to South Africa. He attended a primary school for two years and then returned to Mozambique, where he attended a church school for two years. From the age of sixteen he worked in various places in various capacities. In the 1930s he joined the South African Communist Party. He became a seaman in the Merchant Navy in 1941 and served on a convoy ship during the war. He travelled, or wandered, thereafter for twenty years. During this period it appeared that he began to experience symptoms of psychosis and was hospitalised for short periods in various countries. During a detention on Ellis Island in New York a diagnosis of schizophrenia was eventually made.

In South Africa Tsafendas was classified as white in terms of the country's apartheid system at the time, but was shunned by the white community for being of a darker hue and an outsider. Shortly before the assassination he applied for reclassification from white to coloured to live legally with his mixed-race girlfriend. This was refused.

After the assassination the anti-apartheid movement distanced itself from any association with Tsafendas. Although he is reported to have told the police shortly after the murder that he killed Verwoerd because of his disgust for his racial policies, any political significance that might have been attached to his act of violence was denied to him. At the trial Judge Andries Beyers declared Tsafendas not guilty of murder by reason of insanity. It was claimed by police and his defence that he was inhabited by a giant tapeworm that spoke to him.

Following the trial he was initially accommodated in a cell on death row in Pretoria Central Prison, where he spent the most part of the remainder of his life. When asked in an official enquiry how he was being treated, Tsafendas made no complaint and told the inquiry that he was particularly pleased with the carrots that formed part of his meals. The carrots were good for the tapeworm, he said. He seemed to care for this tapeworm. It was not his enemy.

He was a calm, placid person. There was no prior history of violence and no violent behaviour after the assassination. It appears to have been an isolated and extreme act. He was eventually transferred to Sterkfontein Psychiatric Hospital where he died in 1999 at the age of eighty-one.

To this day it remains unclear what prompted Tsafendas to murder Hendrik Verwoerd. It is uncertain in what ways a lack of any secure attachment in his early years, his restless wanderings around the world and his lack of identity with any community contributed to this one act of appalling violence. It is not known whether the madness of Tsafendas, or the tapeworm, or his alienation from the world, or a sense of political injustice led finally to the assassination.

Yusuf sits quietly during the ward round. He answers my questions in a polite and respectful way. No, he does not understand why he attacked his father. Yes, he understands that it is a terrible thing to have done. No, it will never happen again. Yes, he will take his medication. I am sitting close to him. Under the placid surface he seethes with a violent rage. He is not open to me. I have no understanding of what fuels this. I do not know whether it is his illness, some dark secret in the family, or his rage at the circumstances of his world that make him as dangerous as I think he is.

On the ward he is withdrawn. There is no indication of aggression and no violence. He is passively cooperative with the staff and in his relations with the other patients. Soon I will have to discharge him. He will return home and after a while he will stop taking his medication and it is highly predictable that he will ferociously attack his father again. The father refuses to lay charges against his son, which would enable us to transfer him into the forensic sector. He says his son is sick. He is not a criminal. The father knows the risk. I fear for his life.

There is nothing inherently violent in the nature of mental illness and, more specifically, the psychoses. This misapprehension probably extends to psychiatric hospitals, where violent behaviour might be expected among young men confined involuntarily, but violence is much more likely to occur in emergency units and in the context of intoxication. In the many years I have spent in acute units with predominantly psychotic patients I have never been the victim of a violent assault, nor do I remember fear of any such incident. The widely held assumption that there is an association between mental illness and violence does harm and contributes to the alienation and suffering of those living with mental illnesses. Even in the specific circumstances of command hallucinations, in my clinical experience the voices are more likely to instruct a person to do harm to themselves than to others.

If violence is associated with mental illness it is more likely to be turned against the self than towards others. People living with mental illnesses are more likely to be the victims than the perpetrators of violence.

12

Unreasoned

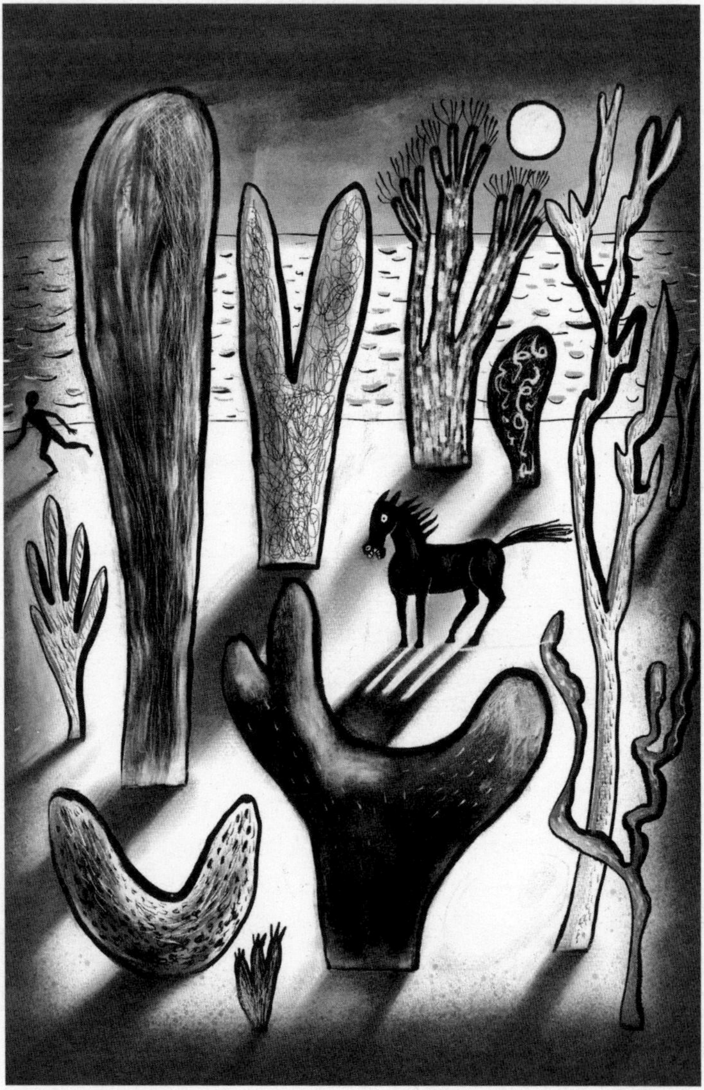

Reason is god. Reason is pure, unsullied by the senses. Reason is what defines us as human, or as superior humans. We proudly identify ourselves as *Homo sapiens*. We aspire to reason. We transcend ourselves through reason, becoming godlike in our emancipation from our awkward contingent selves. Reason is imagined as independent of emotion. We attain the status of civilisation, or simply of ordered civil society, by employing reason to control the disorder and possible chaos of our emotional selves. We have evolved beyond the unreason or lesser consciousness of the lower orders of being to hold notions of power and control, and a moral authority and entitlement to exert this control. We justly benefit from what is due to us through the exercise of the faculty of reason.

This triumphal edifice is dismantled by unreason. Unreason undoes us and we are rendered mad. We become fearful, and cause fear in others, because we imagine that we are less human without reason. We become troubled that the power and authority of reason is illusory or more precarious than we would like to imagine. We are ill at ease with the sense that we are vulnerable, that reason might not protect us from madness. We are unable to console ourselves with the fallacious nonsense that serious mental illness only afflicts those who are in some way morally weak, or fail to use reason to protect themselves.

> Sometimes I am so persistently aware of the curiosity with which I must criticise each moment, as the conversation unwinds, that I must criticise myself out of my presence of mind … so that I lose focus in the crisis … a vague epileptic panic rises … on realising one's own forgetfulness at trying to be lucid … so that I need to keep moving in order to have continuity, as I walk through the silhouetted environment, causing a feeling of calm because of the changing frontiers at the periphery of my vision.

This is one of the many scribbled letters formally addressed to me and shoved under my office door by Govan, a patient I have known for many years and who has remained persistently thought-disordered.

I struggle to make sense of what he is saying. Sometimes I imagine that I might have some inkling of what he is attempting to articulate – and then whatever sense there might be drifts away in a shifting fog of incoherence. Perhaps initially he is describing an excessive form of self-consciousness or self-reflection, to the extent that, with some insight, he 'loses focus'. I am not sure what is meant by 'forgetfulness at trying to be lucid', but it does suggest a struggle for clarity of thought. If he is seeking continuity it is not clear why he should find some calm in the 'changing frontiers', nor why this should be at the periphery of his vision.

Govan is a highly intelligent and very troubled young man. I think he is trying to communicate something very abstract and important to him, but it is not clear. It is not effective. It is convoluted and disorganised, and at some level it seems very possible that he is aware of this, and that must only compound his distress. Perhaps that is why he has to keep moving, as if to be still and be forced to contemplate the disorder of his mind would be intolerable. The calm, he suggests, is ephemeral.

In another letter he writes:

> Dear Dr B. The incongruity of my situation here lies in the normalcy of what is denied as impossible and not the possibility of abnormalcy to which intelligence is applied ... in terms of what goes on and the mystique around my hundred thousand million dollar acquisition ... necessary to provide employment opportunities in terms of landscape gardening the wilderness on Table Mountain so that at least honest labour becomes viable ... so that modernists can terrace and lay drainage with a view to social conservation and crop rotation ... with a view to decentralisation and the restructuring of a global village with parks and orchards in Ruritania ... despite this

grandiose dream I only wish to pursue my personal talents as best I can enjoy them and to plead for the fate of a disorganised global village under the auspices of the United Nations and the World Bank cannot afford bankruptcy. Sincerely, faithfully yours, Govan.

There is again a glimmer of sense in this, and a curious and unexpected insightfulness. He acknowledges the grandiosity of this vaguely articulated scheme, but Table Mountain is oddly relocated in Ruritania, and why the 'modernists' should be responsible for the terracing and drainage is deeply mysterious. Towards the end of the letter, the syntax becomes scrambled. The letter opens and closes with an anomalous formality, and despite or beyond or beneath the disorganisation there is a wistful tone of benevolence, of wanting to make the world a better place.

Adriaan, an older patient whom I have also known for many years, has developed a similar habit of sending me copious numbers of densely scribbled and earnest musings, reflections and complaints. He also stuffs these bewildering missives under my door. Disconcertingly, when I see him in the outpatient clinic he demands to know whether I have studied them, and what I thought, and what he should do. I usually prevaricate in some way; he becomes distracted and to my relief does not pursue his interrogation.

Both Govan and Adriaan write in a way that is for the most part incomprehensible. There are elements at times of coherence but I am not sure whether whatever sense is discerned might be due more to my reconstructing or imagining than what was intended. Regardless of the uncertainty, both of these intelligent and literate patients are communicating in a disorganised manner. This should not obscure their fervent need to explain themselves, to be acknowledged and understood. That is understandable. It is not unreason. In both, there is a clear sense of frustration, of feeling compelled to tell their stories, yet being painfully aware of their inability to do so in an adequate or lucid way.

Marcus tried to explain what was happening to him in another letter of elusive meanings and pained ambivalence:

> Elements of precognitive thoughts overwhelm me. I think I've been born with a psychic link to mankind … I want to use this to grow but it's vexating being bombarded by too many psychic forces … I thought I was capable of producing earthquakes … it's fantastical, it sounds delusional … that I was capable of exerting an influence on the world … I'm not elated by these powers … I just accept it … they have this surveillance, this inner knowledge of me … eventually I align myself … balance out … get back my privacy … with the medication I get more barriers … without treatment I worry more about myself, my whole being becomes painful … people attack me because of my influence … sometimes they don't intentionally do it … it just comes out of them … it's just got to do with humans … it's just the pain of life … I've come to accept it … I'm trying to raise the consciousness of people on earth … I did the striking of the legs and then there were five earthquakes across the world … at the same time I don't create earthquakes unnecessarily … the funny thing about this is that I take it terribly seriously.

Much of this appears to be without reason. What might constitute a necessary earthquake is unfathomable, as is the belief that one might cause an earthquake by 'the striking of the legs'. 'Precognitive thoughts' makes no sense, and attacking others, whether intentionally or not, and being 'just human' is difficult to grasp or needs elaboration to be meaningful.

Much of this is nevertheless clear. Marcus feels that he is under some form of attack, and he is making a strenuous attempt to protect himself. He is both powerful, which he experiences as burdensome, and painfully vulnerable. It is possible but not clear that the one state might compensate for the other. It would be wrong to dismiss these utterances as being entirely without reason. Things surely can be reasonable to a degree, and much might depend on our being willing to understand and to grant meaningfulness.

Biologically, the delusional belief reflects a formulation, at the neocortical level, recruiting often peculiar and deeply personal idioms, of what can only be assumed to be a state of unremitting anguish or noise mediated at lower levels. Owing to the impairment of an abstracting capacity, which is a feature both of schizophrenia and damage to the dorsolateral convexity, this construct is made concrete. It is a solution, yet it is not a solution. Being bombarded by psychic forces provides Marcus with an explanation, but the experience of it is 'vexating'.

The dates are debatable, but evidence from tool-making, cave art and rudimentary musical instruments approximately forty to seventy thousand years ago reflects a capacity to reach beyond the phenomenal world and form alternative representations of reality. This capacity seems to have developed as a function of a critical mass of synaptic or neuronal connectivity in the higher centres of the central nervous system. This seeking of alternative representations does not represent reason. It might be imagined as a yearning beyond reason, beyond the surfaces of our quotidian lives, with a neurological correlate that illustrates the most developed and sophisticated aspects of our embodied and limited selves. Reason, it seems, is not enough. We need something more, perhaps something transcendent and unconfined by reason to grant some necessary meaning to our lives. That need seems to be something quite fundamentally human, whether or not we are considered mad.

Some months ago I was gazing in perplexed wonder at a Rothko in the National Gallery in London. The painting was entirely abstract. It was devoid of any representational references and the colours were sombre. I have no understanding of what drew me to this painting nor what moved me about it. There is no reason in it at all, but it would be ridiculous to conclude that this might diminish or undermine the mysterious power that the painting held over me.

Regarding reason and unreason in a simplistic binary relationship – that something is either reasonable or not reasonable, without any murky, intermediate degrees of reasonableness – makes little sense and has damaging consequences with regard to how we understand and treat mental illness.

Madness is in part defined by unreason, its expressions causing fear and exclusion through being un-understandable and inexplicable. Being more sceptical of the worship of reason, being a little more aware of the tenuous role that reason plays in much of our lives, might then incline us less to consider the mad as being other and dispose us more to inclusivity.

We live, for the most part, probably by unreason. We are sustained by our desires, which are without reason, and we cope with life through an understandable yet unreasonable refusal of our mortality or a denial of its certainty. It is strange to fear unreason when it seems to govern so much of what we feel and think and do.

13

Wonder

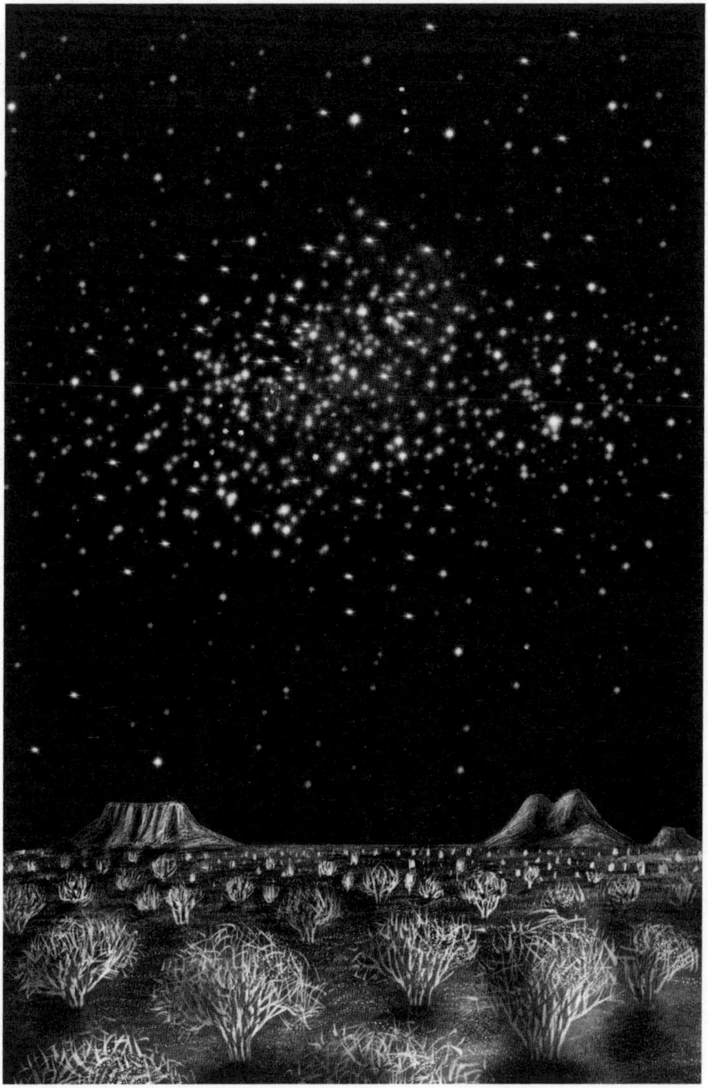

We are sitting in a circle in the ward-round room. It is a Wednesday afternoon and we are discussing the new admissions. Renos was brought in during the latter part of last week. At the time of his admission his behaviour was chaotic and aggressive, but according to the nursing reports he settled fairly rapidly. We make an effort to see all the new patients. It is partly to introduce ourselves and to explain the procedures of the ward, but also hopefully an attempt to put them at their ease in very difficult and often bewildering circumstances.

Renos is remarkably relaxed. He seems quite bizarrely content. I ask him how the weekend was, a ridiculous question as it could only have been miserable. He had been confined throughout in a closed, very noisy and probably frightening ward. He beams, to our great surprise, and declares that he has had a most wonderful weekend. We enquire tentatively how this could have been possible in such difficult circumstances. Again he smiles broadly and with some pride points to his fashionable and expensive running shoes. He indicates a coloured disc on the side of the shoe which I think enables one to adjust the pressure in the shoe's heel. 'You see, Doctor, all I have to do is press this button, which is what I did on Friday night, and whoosh, I am flown to the moon. It was a fantastic flight, and guess what, who should be waiting for me on the moon? It was Beyoncé! She was stark naked! She was so excited to see me. We made the most incredible love throughout the night. She wouldn't leave me alone. I was exhausted. Finally, when it had almost become too much for me, I said goodbye and thanked her for this most wonderful adventure. I pressed the button again on my shoe, and whoosh, I was back in the ward. I am not complaining. I need the rest. It was amazing, fantastic!' He leans back in his chair, it seems to us in a state of blissful satiation, and yawns. 'Wow,' he sighs happily, gazing around at his astonished audience. 'Wow, all you good people. What a fabulous weekend.'

A medical student is struggling to suppress her laughter. The rest of us are nodding earnestly, trying to decide how to respond appropriately to this strange and rather wonderful story.

A caution is necessary in merely considering the notion of wonder in regard to madness. Wonder might be considered romantic, and in this way undermine the gravity of mental illness. It might lure us into complacency in that, if there is some wonder, things cannot be too bad – or that treatment is then either misguided or unnecessary. Yet it seems sad and rather impoverished not to acknowledge the strange wonder of these stories. This becomes even more of an issue if these idiosyncratic narratives, confabulations or delusions, or however they might be labelled, are construed as a struggle on the part of our patients to give some form and meaning to what might otherwise be experienced as intolerable noise. Renos is admitted against his will to a chaotic ward. He is frightened. He has to get away. He flies to the moon where he has a prolonged erotic encounter with a world-renowned pop star. He flies back willingly to the hospital. It's very curious, but it is one way of coping. Certainly, it has done nobody any harm. On the contrary, it seems to have given him a great deal of pleasure.

I am attending a meeting in the ward when a commotion arises. This meeting is rather oddly called a 'climate' meeting, the idea being that I and the nursing staff sit in a circle with the patients and listen to whatever issues they want to raise. This is a fairly formal, regimented event, the nurse in charge allowing only one patient to speak at a time and limiting his time to a few minutes. But on this occasion any semblance of order dramatically breaks down. One young man, Tswalo, begins to shriek and howl. He grasps his abdomen as if in severe bouts of pain. To everybody's amazement it appears that this young man believes he is in labour. He falls to the ground and writhes about. The other patients mill around, initially bewildered by what is going on. Then they decide to take action.

They become purposefully engaged, one running to get wet towels, others attempting to soothe and comfort the now terrified Tswalo. The nurses stand back, bemused. This goes on for a while. Each patient is occupied with some helpful task. Nobody laughs. Nobody is impatient or angered by this extraordinary performance. The pain increases, the wailing and shrieking reach a crescendo, and then parturition appears to take place. I have no idea what is going on as the patients are now huddled over Tswalo, who is lying on his back weeping. They are stroking and comforting him, and two take a dirty bundle of rags away from him. Eventually calm ensues. Everybody seems exhausted by these dramatic events but there is an atmosphere of excitement and celebration. Tswalo regains his composure and manages to get back onto his feet.

I am about to leave the ward when he approaches me with the dirty bundle cradled in his arms. He is smiling coyly and seems proud. The other patients gather around him, making cooing noises. It is clearly my duty as the doctor on the ward to admire whatever he has produced. Wrapped in the rags is a pair of dirty shoes. I have no idea how to respond; this is not part of one's training as a medical student, nor as a specialist in psychiatry. I make what I hope is some sort of positive, affirmative response, but I certainly cannot match the enthusiasm of the patients who attended to him. I leave the ward a happy place.

What might have prompted Tswalo to believe that he was in labour is a complete mystery, and I imagine that no amount of psychoanalytical investigation will make it less so. He is a robust young Xhosa man. He showed no indication on the ward that he might think that he was a woman, let alone a pregnant woman. The labour and the birth of the shoes was a surprise to all of us, but what was perhaps more of a surprise to me was the engagement and the kindness of the other patients. It seemed genuine. I did not form the impression that they might have been bored and welcomed the distraction. I did not sense that they were amusing themselves by participating in an absurd charade. They wanted to help the young man. They wanted to comfort him and get him through the crisis, although they must have been as mystified as I was by his behaviour.

It seems important to me to acknowledge this kindness, which seems quite wonderful, beyond the strange and at times frightening behaviours associated with madness. The kindness is not madness. It might be a special kind of kindness, recognising that somebody is mad, or behaving madly, and yet is in distress and is in need of care and attention. It is all the more remarkable and moving that this kindness came from a group of very troubled and frightened young men who were struggling to cope with their own psychotic demons.

James and Justin are two cousins whom I see every month in the outpatient clinic. Their stories are sad, even tragic, and yet the dignified way in which they both cope with their illness fills me with wonder. James was working on a doctoral degree in nuclear physics when things started to go awry and then fall apart. It is not clear whether it was the stress of his academic work, perhaps, or a strong family history of schizophrenia that led to this collapse. In all likelihood it was a combination of factors. An admission to our unit was required and there was a fairly prolonged struggle to gain control of his symptoms. He regained a degree of equanimity but he never fully recovered. His studies were suspended but eventually it became clear that he would never be able to complete the doctorate. He had become disabled to the extent that he would probably never be able to work again, or not in a way that would enable him to live independently. He became dependent on his parents, a father who suffered from a severe degenerative neuromuscular disorder and a mother living with schizophrenia, both of whom had held high hopes for their brilliant son.

When I see James in the outpatient clinic he is dishevelled and, although it is a hot summer's day, he is wearing a woollen cap and a thick jersey. His hair is uncombed and lanky, his teeth are black and his clothes are untidy and unwashed. I am with a group of undergraduate students.

He greets us enthusiastically and insists on learning each of their names. I ask him whether he is comfortable with their being with us for the meeting. He responds that he loves being with the students.

From a duffel bag he brings out a number of pamphlets that he proudly distributes. He tells us that they are an explanation of his philosophy that seeks to integrate physics with religion. He tells us that he has sent these documents to his former professor at the university, and also to the pope, the queen of England and the president of the United States of America. He is delighted to have received a card from the pope. It is a photograph of His Excellency and a short homily, something that is presumably dispatched to all those who presume to communicate with the holy man. From his professor he has received a rather curt and dismissive letter; from the queen and the American president he has received nothing.

He is undaunted. He is joyfully unfazed by these negative responses to what he regards as his life's work. Their affirmation is not that important to him. He will not be deterred from his mission. The students are most welcome to study his pamphlets but he quite understands if they do not. He knows they are much occupied with their studies, that they might feel overwhelmed, and he acknowledges that his grand ideas might not be considered relevant to their medical curriculum. He is considerate and animated and elated. When the meeting ends he thanks us all profusely for the attention we have shown him. He says he looks forward to the next meeting in a month's time.

The students have just started their four-week block in psychiatry. I don't know what they were expecting but they seem surprised and charmed. They wonder how they would cope in his circumstances, and think that, in all probability, they would feel profoundly disappointed and angry and resentful and depressed and hopeless. They wonder at his exuberant resilience. He is obviously damaged, having suffered severe losses, but he seems to us quite heroically undefeated.

His cousin Justin comes in after him. He is much better kempt than

James and his demeanour is courteous and rather formal. He lacks James's excited intensity and seems more cautious and reserved. He also had his first psychotic breakdown at university, while studying philosophy, but quite remarkably recovered to the extent that he was able to resume his studies and eventually gain a bachelor's degree. He also politely asks the students their names and enquires about their backgrounds. He even manages a few words in isiXhosa, clearly in an attempt to put them at ease. He is gentle and kind. It is not how the students are used to being treated by patients outside the field of psychiatry. They are more accustomed to being regarded with disdain and impatience; their presence in clinical encounters is often resented.

Justin enquires earnestly about my well-being and that of my young daughters, as he always does. I am not sure why I answer him on this occasion in the way I do – perhaps it is to indicate to him that I register his concern and do not dismiss it as mere politeness. Ridiculously, I tell him that one of my daughters was in a state of some distress that morning because her cat had eaten her pet mouse. He appears to ponder this and then says, 'The cat will now become all the more loved because the mouse is inside her.'

He is proposing a strange but also creative strategy to console my daughter. Rather than considering this unfortunate event as an act of gratuitous violence on the part of the cat, he is suggesting to us a sort of two-for-the-price-of-one deal in that the mouse is not gone, but incorporated into the cat. The mouse has not been subtracted, but added to the cat. In his kind, albeit rather peculiar way, he is trying to help. Another patient might quite understandably have said, 'What on earth has your daughter's pet saga got to do with my predicament?' Justin is reaching out.

This is not the characteristic behaviour associated with schizophrenia, often described as autistic, whereby patients turn inwards and become remote and inaccessible. Perhaps it is inevitable that generalisations are made, that we think in terms of stereotypes, but it does harm. People are not schizophrenic. That is offensive and stigmatising. People might live with or suffer from schizophrenia. We would surely be outraged if somebody was described as cancerous, or tuberculous. Suffering is personal and subjective. Making a strenuous effort not to treat any patients as being the same might go some way, at least, to mitigating the alienation and exclusion that is so much part of the suffering of the mentally ill. In the same way, regarding schizophrenia or psychosis or madness in an irredeemably bleak light is not helpful. There must be some hope and wonder to sustain us all.

There is another element of wonder in this domain that is seldom acknowledged. On many occasions I have thought recovery unimaginable. These young men seemed so immersed in their madness, their symptoms so pervasive and intractable, that any way of retrieving them seemed impossible. Witnessing, even after a few days, the faltering steps out of madness, the smile, the restoration of spontaneity and of the self, was profoundly moving – and on many occasions inspiring. The perception that mental illness cannot be treated effectively is wrong and harmful. Many factors contribute to this perception. Principally perhaps is the notion of treatment as curative. The great majority of illnesses, particularly of a chronic nature such as diabetes or cardiovascular disease or cancer, are not amenable to cure, but can certainly be successfully treated or managed. This also applies to most mental illnesses. Hopelessness and resignation are not appropriate and can only compound suffering. Wonder is defiant and restorative.

Our team is gathered again in a ward-round room, on this occasion in the pre-discharge ward. Kgabu is ushered in by a nurse. He has a formal, dignified, authoritative demeanour. I introduce myself and the members of the team, and ask him how he is coping. He says he is doing very well, thank you, and enquires about my own well-being. I thank him in turn for his concern and then ask him about the circumstances leading to his admission to the hospital. He seems surprised, and says, 'But I am the doctor in charge here. I am the consultant.' We are all taken aback. I then ask rather hesitantly where that might put me, being under the impression that I am the doctor in charge. He seems to think carefully about this, then answers solemnly: 'You, Dr B – you are the Master of the Universe.'

This indicates that, although in a rather grand way, he has some sense of a hierarchy operating in the unit – but more importantly it reflects a dissatisfaction with the passive role of a patient as a recipient of care and the wish to fulfil a role that he imagines is more helpful. It also makes my day.

A sense of wonder is not indulgently romantic or sentimental, but necessary. It does not diminish the tragedy of severe mental illness. We need to attend to the stories our patients tell us. We need to acknowledge the strange wonderfulness of these accounts, and the wonder of resilience in circumstances of extreme adversity, and the wonder, sometimes, of recovery.

14

Shame

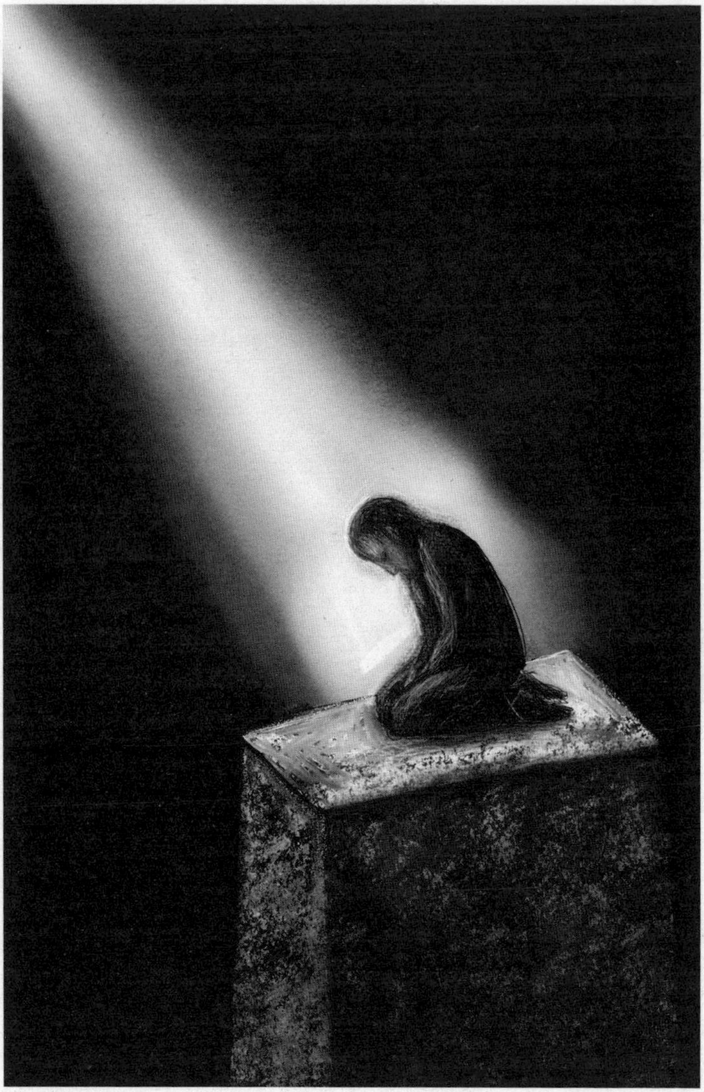

Mental illness is shameful. Suicide and attempted suicide are shameful acts. It is dismaying and perplexing why extremes of human suffering should be considered shameful.

The shame might be personal. It might be felt by the family of somebody afflicted with mental illness. It might be the shame of a community for not doing more, and it might be the shame upon government for the neglect of, and in recent events a criminal and callous disregard for the mentally ill. It might be the shame we all feel, to some extent, for not understanding or not being able to help.

The personal shame is the saddest. It is profoundly wrong that somebody struggling with thoughts and feelings that are unbidden and tormenting should be further burdened by a sense of shame. This shame has many elements, a number of which hover at the edges of consciousness or emanate vaguely from cultural beliefs to which one might not subscribe, yet which exert a pervasive and subliminal influence.

I might call myself an atheist but believe or sense in some way that it is wrong to kill myself. A precept might be more explicit. The Koran is emphatic that suicide is sinful, and curiously will be punished by everlasting torment in hell. My aunt committed suicide in a postpartum psychotic depression. She was a Catholic; because of the manner of her shameful death she was buried in unconsecrated ground. In this context mental illness has no meaning. It provides no explanation. It is irrelevant. Suicide is sinful. It is shameful. It is taking away from God what belongs to God.

Mental illness in these realms of dogma is a frail construct. It cannot account for or excuse this terrible sin of theft from the almighty. Part of this must be a fear that is part of the human condition. If there is no God who cares for us, for whom it matters whether we kill ourselves or not, what is there? An indifferent god is intolerable, and if he or she does not care, what are the grounds for leading a moral life, or what is the purpose of anything at all? If we are so terribly free, we are at liberty to kill ourselves, and for many this is abhorrent and shameful.

This persists beyond religion, but perhaps in a more attenuated or insidious way. There is a kind of faith in secular humanism, but it is not overt. The notion of shame is less explicit, or it is unacceptable because of its religious connotations. The faith or the belief is in our humanity. Associated with this is the belief that we, and not God, are in control of our destinies. We exert free will. We have freedom of choice. We hold responsibility for the choices we make in our lives. The self is central. It is holy. We cannot blame God or fate when things go wrong. In this context, mental illness – or more specifically psychotic states – are confounding. There is a loss of the sense that one is in control of one's thoughts and actions. The notion of the self becomes tenuous and disintegrates. In this respect one loses one's humanity. Shame is not invoked, but it might be felt. Mental illness is an abstraction. It is too vague and precarious a notion to account for this profoundly altered state of being.

It seems possible that these implicit ways of thinking at least to some extent might account for the bewildering persistence of stigma, or the casting of the mentally ill as other, beyond the fold of humanity.

Allied to this is a faith or an assumption that, as we are in control of our lives, it is our duty to take responsibility for how we choose to lead our lives. This is undeniable. It is fundamental to who we are. To think otherwise is to deny our humanity. If it is not shameful, it is unimaginable.

Eusebius has been struggling with schizophrenia for years. For the moment it is contained. He attends the outpatient clinic regularly. He takes the prescribed medication. He lives in a group home and sees his family on the weekends. He is coping, he says, but it is difficult. He is well enough to know that he is not well. He has to live with the past and he is unsure about the future. He is not at all certain that he is strong enough to stay as he is at present. The illness is too unpredictable. It is too much for him. He cannot undo what has happened. He is ashamed, and that further burdens him.

When he was ill he assaulted his mother. He cannot understand how he could have done this. It was as if it was not him, he says, but it was him and he cannot make sense of it. Can madness undo you in this way? What strange illness is this that makes you not yourself? He was running naked in the streets. He was shrieking at strangers. People try to reassure him. They say it was just the illness. He must not be ashamed. He was not himself. He was not responsible for what he did. He will be all right. He must just be careful.

Eusebius does not really understand what that means. Deep down, he believes that this madness is part of who he is and will never go away. He is humiliated. He is unworthy of self-respect. He is grateful to those who try to comfort him. He nods politely and says, 'Yes, I understand, it is just an illness, like diabetes perhaps, and it can be controlled, and it does not have to ruin my life,' but I sense that he does not believe this is true.

He is not like the others. His friends from his school years have moved on. Some have already graduated from university. He has been left behind. A bright future has been taken away from him. He wanted to be an architect. Now that seems impossible. There is little or no prospect of his being able to work in a way that will make him independent of his family. He attends an art class and he does beading but he finds it extremely awkward. He is confronted with his disability. He is shamefully unproductive. He has failed.

When he visits his mother he does not know whether it is in his imagination but he thinks he sees fear in her eyes. She cannot forget what he did to her. He cannot live like this and so he stops his medication and within weeks he is back in our wards, ranting and raving, behaving in a wild and dangerous way that will only cause him further embarrassment when he recovers. He is trapped in his illness. For him, madness is a transient and illusory escape that only causes further hurt and shame.

Johannes has recovered from a manic episode of a bipolar mood disorder. He is ambivalent about these episodes. In some respects, he tells me, he thrives on the mania. He says it is the best feeling possible.

He would not wish it away. He is filled with energy and everything is possible. On this occasion he visited a nightclub with a friend. He became intoxicated. He bought drinks for strangers, groped at the dancers and fought with the bouncers, who eventually tried to evict him. He ended the night in a police cell and his daughter was summoned the next day. It would all have been hilarious, he says, if not for the reproach and the anger he saw in his daughter's eyes when she came to collect him. She said she was ashamed of him, and this had hurt him deeply. For this reason he says he will now act responsibly and take his medication diligently. His wife left him years earlier because of his wayward and reckless behaviour. He could not allow himself to alienate his daughter. He appears to be contrite. He says childishly, 'I am going to be a good boy.' I am not at all confident. I am not sure whether the sense of shame is sufficiently strong for him to be able to put aside the raptures of his mania.

Henri is profoundly depressed. He says he has recovered to some extent. He no longer feels hopeless. There is some vague glimmer of a future. He is no longer hell-bent on ending his life. He says he can see things more clearly now, but that means that he can see that he has failed his family, that he is a worthless husband and father to his long-suffering wife and children. In one way these sentiments are part of his depressive illness, but in another this appraisal is valid and understandable. He has lost his job. His colleagues said the company could no longer afford the many days he took off work because he said he could no longer cope. He started to drink heavily. He resisted the increasingly desperate attempts of his friends and family to reach out to him. Then one morning he told his wife that he was taking the car out for a drive, to try to sort himself out, he said. She became suspicious and went to look for him. She found him barely conscious in the garage with a pipe leading from the exhaust into the car, where he sat slumped in the driver's seat. He was resuscitated and there were no adverse effects, other than shame. This is the worst part of it, he says, and he does not see how it will ever go away.

He also believes, and I think with reason, that his family is ashamed because of what he has done. His wife is religious, and although she is not devout it seems very probable that she believes that his attempted suicide was a sinful act. She might seek to lessen the burden by saying to me and to her husband that she accepts that he has been suffering from some sort of malady, but I don't think she believes it and I think his desperate act lies heavily on the marriage. She tells me that she also feels ashamed that she has not been able to help him. Shame confuses and complicates his depression, and is not something that a pill will take away.

I find it difficult to say to a family that there is no explanation. I sense that they feel there has to be. Where does this madness come from? There has to be an explanation, an answer. Perhaps if there is a known cause, there is a solution. I do not think it is helpful to assert causation when the circumstances are most often fraught with uncertainty. Invoking a genetic contribution, for example, or environmental stressors can itself too easily lead to self-recrimination and self-blame and then shame. If schizophrenia is an illness like diabetes or tuberculosis, there has to be a cause, as there are known causes of these illnesses. If there are no known causes, we will invent causes: the bad genes or the bad upbringing, or devil possession or an evil spirit or a bad spell or punishment for some transgression. Even if we are able to come to terms with the uncertainties about why a psychosis might develop, we carry the burden of what we imagine our families and communities are thinking: 'They must have done something wrong. These things don't just come from nowhere.'

There is another cause of shame with regard to mental illness, and this pertains to neglect. This manifests in many ways, including the low priority accorded to psychiatric services despite the great burden represented by mental illness on the community, in terms of both human suffering and economic losses. This neglect recently reached a grotesque nadir in the deaths of over a hundred patients in the Gauteng province of South Africa. These extremely vulnerable people were removed from private health-care provider Life Esidimeni to unsupervised care in community establishments, where they died from a range of preventable causes. This cynical and criminal disregard for human life is a disgrace to the elected government, and we are all deeply affected by the shame of what has been allowed to happen in our midst. It is difficult not to imagine, in this atrocious circumstance, that the lives of those living with mental illnesses are considered less worthy, and in this respect we are all diminished.

To believe, through fear or ignorance, that mental illness is in any way shameful is wrong. It causes further suffering and it is as offensive as it is shameful.

15

The dream of the community

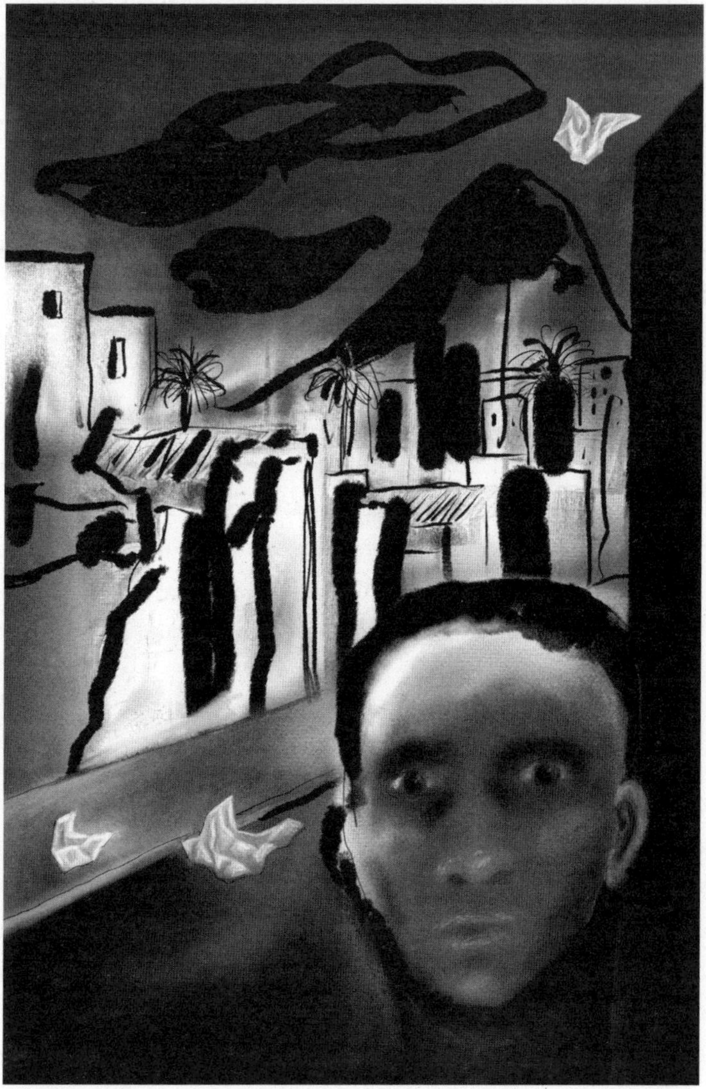

Over ninety are now dead. There is concern that this number is likely to rise. Many remain missing. For some there are no records. It is not known whether they are dead or alive. They have just disappeared. The health ombudsman has found that the most common cause of the deaths was pneumonia, followed by uncontrolled seizures. All but one of these deaths are considered to have been preventable. Extremely vulnerable people have died for lack of care. On average, patients died within two months of the transfer from the Life Healthcare Group's Life Esidimeni to a range of non-regulated 'care homes'. 'Esidimeni' means 'place of dignity'. The reasons for the transfer are given by the responsible health official as 'cost containment'.

This is the number of deaths that took place between 23 March and 19 December 2016. The most recent estimate is that one hundred and forty four patients in total died. Patients were found to be starving and dehydrated. Relatives testify that the patients had been given no extra blankets and warm clothing during the harsh winter. There are reports of patients being left naked and chained to beds without mattresses and next to dead bodies. There are reports of physical and sexual abuse, of cruel and inhumane treatment. Twenty deaths occurred in an unlicensed care and rehabilitation centre named Precious Angels.

This calamity occurred following a decision on the part of the Department of Health to terminate the contract with Life Esidimeni Health Care Centre in the province of Gauteng and to transfer patients with mental-health problems to a range of non-licensed non-governmental organisations throughout the province. An estimated one thousand three hundred and seventy chronically ill patients were transferred from 1 June to 30 June in what was described as a chaotic and shambolic process. The contract was terminated to save money. State-subsidised patients were to be moved from the private hospital group to the care of cheaper community-based organisations. The health official responsible for this decision persisted with the plan despite opposition from families, health-care experts and activists, who warned that these community organisations were not able to provide the high-level care that the patients needed. The aim was to save the province R320 per patient per day. The assumption was that the professional care needed by these patients could be provided by non-governmental organisations for R100 per day.

The *Report into the Circumstances Surrounding the Deaths of Mentally Ill Patients: Gauteng Province*, requested by the Minister of Health, found evidence of human-rights violations. There had been a total disregard of the rights of the patients and their families – including, among many others, the right to human dignity, the rights to life, and the rights to freedom and security of persons. Negligent and reckless decisions and actions included grossly inadequate preparation for the transfer, the transfer of patients without the knowledge of their families, the transfer of patients to distant locations, overcrowding at community centres that were unlicensed and unregulated, a lack of provision for community health-care services, a lack of suitably qualified staff at the centres, and the 'precipitous and chaotic' transfer against the advice of experts and mental-health-care practitioners. The manner, the rate, the scale and the speed of transferring such large numbers of vulnerable patients had been reckless. All these decisions and actions ran contrary to governmental policies and strategies of deinstitutionalisation.

A number of recommendations were made. Disciplinary proceedings should be instituted against the officials responsible for gross misconduct and incompetence. The national Minister of Health should request the South African Human Rights Commission to undertake a systematic review of human-rights compliance and possible violations, nationally, related to mental health. Appropriate legal action should be taken against non-governmental organisations found to have been operating unlawfully and where patients died. The national Department of Health should review all non-governmental organisations involved in the project, and those that do not meet the necessary health-care standards should be deregistered and closed down.

Bewilderment and outrage have ensued. There has been a struggle to find the right words to reach a sufficient pitch of indignation and anger that might possibly be considered an appropriate response to these events. Words such as 'tragedy' and 'murder' have been invoked. Neither seems appropriate. Tragedy suggests a degree of inevitability, a misfortune that befalls us and that is beyond our control. This most emphatically does not apply to those who died following the termination of the Life Esidimeni contract. These people died because of incompetence and neglect, but they were not murdered. I do not think there is any evidence of intent. Murder can only be understood in this context as a criminal disregard for the humanity and the lives of others.

We are confounded. We are horrified. We are ashamed. Amid this clamour, perhaps two points need emphasis. It is difficult not to imagine that such a degree of callous indifference on the part of the officials involved could have arisen from a certain attitude towards the mentally ill. None of those making these atrocious decisions were health-care practitioners. They were bureaucrats and politicians. A terrible confusion of incompetence and avarice and an abysmal failure of imagination seem to have led to a collapse of the most basic humanitarian attitudes. It appears that people with mental illnesses are not quite human. They are not deserving of care and respect. They are mere items of cost. They are a burden to society. They are dispensable. If things go wrong, nobody will care too much. We will have achieved the necessary savings. We will have pleased our political masters.

Another profoundly sad and perhaps contentious argument is that, although these decisions and actions represent a grotesque extreme, they should not be regarded as exceptional. It is not rare nor does it cause an outcry that people with serious mental illnesses are neglected and abandoned in the community. As a result there is further suffering. There is exclusion and ostracisation and this might extend in many parts of the world to persecution and demonisation. Simple lack of basic care might lead to early death but for the most part this goes unnoticed. We want to believe in the community. We need to believe in care in the community. What has happened here is intolerable. Anger and indignation is of little import if it does not compel us to learn some painful and profoundly disconcerting lessons from these appalling events.

We are about to discharge Mashile and it fills me with foreboding. I don't know how long it will last. His family share these concerns. They also fear for their own safety. When we discharged him previously things fell apart rapidly. Both parents work. There is nobody at home to care for Mashile during the day. There is no day centre in the vicinity. He is vulnerable. Gangsters have followed him home from the clinic before, pretending to befriend him and persuading him to part with a portion of his disability grant to procure drugs. When the parents returned home, the gangsters were there. They threatened the family with violence if any attempt was made to call the police. It amused them to watch Mashile become intoxicated and then psychotic after using cannabis. They drifted away after he was readmitted to hospital, but the parents knew they would be waiting. They would find him again at the clinic when he went to collect his medication or at the welfare centre where he needed to collect his grant money. They would follow him home again and intimidate the family and use their drugs with impunity. Mashile would get sick again and require readmission.

This is all so predictable: 'We are all in danger now, so why, Doctor, don't you keep him? You know he will be back within months, maybe weeks, if he manages to stay alive, if the gangsters don't kill him for his grant.' The parents know this appeal is hopeless. We have been through this before. I have told them that I cannot keep him in hospital if he has recovered and he is well. We need the bed for those, many like Mashile, who have yet again broken down for lack of care in the community. We cannot use our very limited psychiatric services to treat the historical and socioeconomic ills of the city, and perhaps most importantly Mashile wants to go. He says he is better and wants his freedom.

The exasperated parents ask what sort of freedom this is, to be abused and exploited by others. When I say we do not have the right to keep him against his will they become angry and ask: do they not also have rights, the right to feel safe in their own home and to the peace of mind that their son is safe and being cared for? They see no end to this. It is a miserable session and it ends with a very clear sense on the part of the parents, but also on my own part, of dissatisfaction and frustration owing to the limitations of what we can and cannot do. I feel that we are failing this family – not because we are refusing to keep their son in hospital, but because of the woeful inadequacies of the provision of care in the community.

Political and economic and ideological issues are confounded by the various terms adopted to pursue different agendas. This is apart from ethical concerns and arguments about what might constitute optimal care. Community care is not the opposite of hospital care. Hospitalisation is not institutionalisation. There is a persisting misapprehension that an admission to a specialist psychiatric hospital means being 'put away', and that this is of indefinite duration. This is a reflection of the past, in most countries of the world; in present times, it is indefensible.

A combination of factors, including changes in attitude and psychopharmacological advances, render any notion of institutionalisation or incarceration redundant and unethical. Yet to this day people, possibly squeamish about using the word 'patient' as a demeaning epithet, choose the more offensive term 'inmate', conjuring up, however unintentionally, the sinister and persisting fear of the asylum.

In the hospital where I work, the average length of stay is four weeks. Some patients do stay longer, but the reason for this is most often the absence of a suitable place in the community. 'Care in the community' is a fraught term and is laden with aspirational and ideological freight. Whatever we might wish to believe, care in the community too often translates into neglect and abandonment, homelessness, and incarceration – not in hospitals, but in prisons. This most emphatically cannot be used as an argument against community care for people with severe mental illnesses. It does require the abandonment of any notion that this might be a cost-saving exercise and of an entirely cynical attitude that, without the provision of the necessary resources, neglect and a new form of exclusion can be presented as a progressive policy.

In the best of all possible worlds, plans are made for Mashile's discharge from hospital. He is referred to a day centre, which he will attend immediately following his discharge. There he will be assessed in terms of his needs, not his disabilities. He will perhaps join a pottery class and start some basic training in carpentry. He will be part of a group who understand and support each other. He will be introduced to the community nurse who will supervise his care but most importantly provide further support and encouragement. Should he perhaps develop troubling side-effects of his medication, the community health-care worker will discuss this with the supervising psychiatrist and the necessary changes will be made without Mashile having to wait for hours in a hospital outpatient clinic for a hasty consultation with a psychiatrist to whom he is a stranger. His parents are able to relax, knowing that he is safe during the day. He begins to show an aptitude for carpentry and is invited to join a workshop where he will earn a small income to supplement his disability grant. He takes great pride in his achievements. He is valued by others at the day centre but also by members of the community who see in him no reason to fear those who live with psychotic disorders. His days have purpose and meaning.

There is no justification for abandoning what might at present be dismissed as a wishful fantasy. Beyond the allocation of resources, beyond mere tolerance, a fundamental change in thinking is required. It is not simply to be unafraid of otherness – it is to seek it out and attach value to otherness and in this way to extend ourselves and assert our humanity. It is to refuse the uniformity imposed upon us by the marketplace, the inherited and learnt definition of ourselves that shapes our attitudes in so many subtle and insidious ways. We need to be willing to accept the need for change in the way we see ourselves and the way we behave towards others.

Life Esidimeni has shamed us all. Perhaps especially in this divided and fractured country we need urgently to extend and complicate our lives by engaging with otherness, rather than retreating into familiar territories that can no longer be consoling: the precarious and absurd identities of race and nationality and normality or sanity. It is surely not impossible to imagine that we might be more free if we were to extricate ourselves from the suburbs and fortresses of our fear. It is a dream that otherness might be not a source of anxiety and dread but a source of wonder, and it is regrettable that so many of us seem resigned to this being merely a dream.

16

The status of disability and its complications

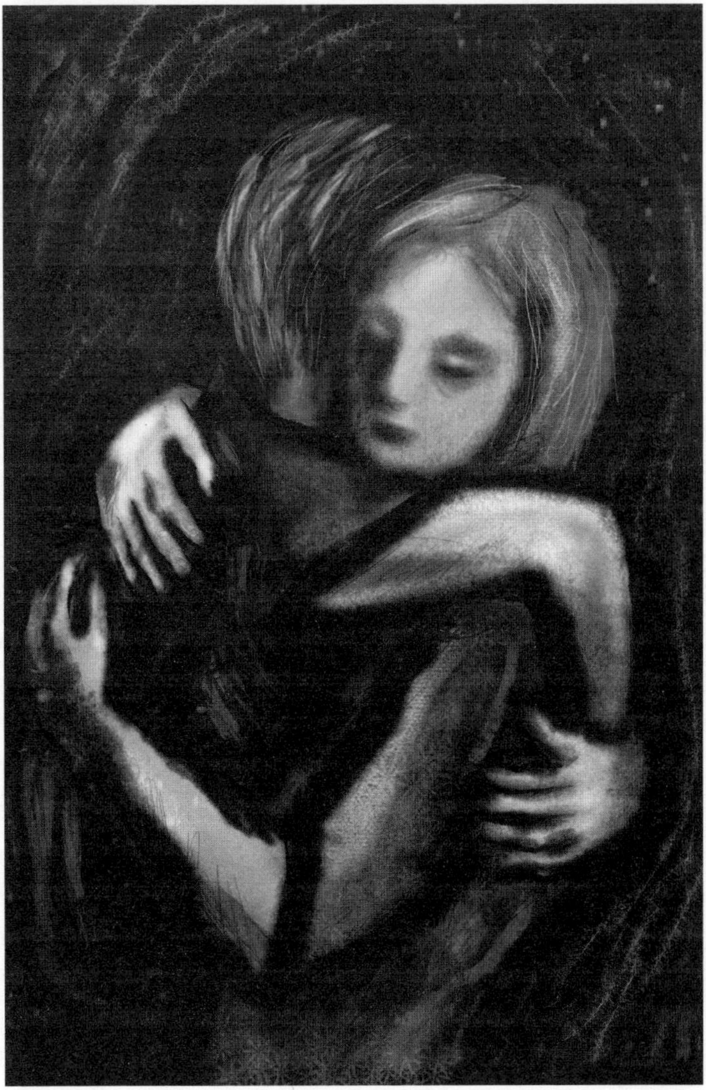

Hannes stares at me vacantly. He is sitting slumped in a chair in the outpatient clinic. I don't think he wants to be here but on the other hand I don't know where he would rather be. He appears to be disinterested in my questions. He is fine, he says. There are no problems. No, there is nothing he wants to raise with me. He stares through the window at the birds on the river. He sighs and shrugs. He is impatient. He is ill at ease. The only reason he is here is for me to sign the application for the renewal of his disability grant. The rest is just noise, a tiresome formality.

I persist and clearly it annoys him. I want to know how he spends his days. I want to know what occupies him. When he wakes in the morning, what does he think? What does he hope for? I suppose what I want to know is what gives meaning and value to his life. I suspect the answer to this is that nothing gives meaning and value to his life. These issues are meaningless to him. He drifts along, he gets by. I am not to burden him with these irrelevant concerns.

But why not do something, I ask, anything, however small or insignificant it might seem, just to make it worth his while to get up in the morning, just to have something maybe to look forward to? He is impassive. 'I am not bored,' he says. I tell him, or I try to reassure him, that I am not suggesting that he go out and seek some kind of formal employment. I know that he is afraid that any kind of work will jeopardise the disability grant. I also know that his finding any kind of paid work is almost impossible. He has no skills, no experience and most importantly no motivation. Yet anything to give him at least some purpose and direction in life I imagine would be helpful. Maybe he could develop some skill, he could learn to cook, he could take drawing classes, maybe he could learn a new language. He looks at me as if I am the patient, as if I am mad. I am making no sense. Why don't I just get off his back and sign the wretched form?

I want to say that I acknowledge that he is disabled, but not so disabled. It is difficult to find the right language and all the more difficult because he is not interested. It is as if this designation of being disabled has seeped into him and has disabled him at some deeper level.

In another societal domain, being identified as disabled can carry with it the added burden of stigmatisation. As I am writing this, a report emerges in the media concerning difficulties encountered by those trying to provide help for disabled children. A project manager at the Tshwaranang District Project Centre in a rural area of Limpopo expresses the concern that beliefs linking witchcraft to disabled persons are problematic, and that one of the major obstacles to obtaining the limited help that is available is stigmatisation. She reports: 'There are those who still believe that if you are disabled you are cursed and bewitched. And so we see parents trying to hide their disabled children.' Injustice is laid on misfortune: not only are you disabled, but you are believed to be cursed and prevented from getting the support and help you need.

The burden of disability in this harsh world is compounded by exclusion. Hannes is extremely vulnerable. One aspect of the schizophrenia he is living with is a loss of drive or volition. This is associated with a precarious sense of self and agency. There is a danger that one's own perception of disability can compound the disability. A special effort is required to encourage somebody struggling with schizophrenia to believe in their self-worth and regain control of their lives. It is not going to be possible if the parents of the disabled child believe that he or she is bewitched. This most unfortunate child would be all too likely to believe this too.

It is difficult and unlikely (although not impossible) that these issues will be attended to in the turmoil of an admission ward or in the outpatient clinic or community clinic, with a restless queue of patients waiting to be seen. It is important, it is necessary, but perhaps most often it seems too much or is too uncertain whether the effort expended might result in the elusive reward of somebody regaining a sense of purpose and hope. The more likely response – and I do not think this is confined to the local situation – is a hastily written script and a renewed application for the provision of a disability grant. Sadly, I think very many of us give up too soon on any expectation that our patients will recover.

This is not in any way an argument against the notion of disability itself, and certainly not against the desperate need for the provision of disability grants. It is an expression of concern about some of the ramifications and unintended consequences of invoking disability. Identifying disability, recognising its extent and the burden it exerts on individuals, their families, on health services and the economy, is of great importance for many reasons. It provides for the allocation of necessary resources and services. It should (but does not necessarily) stimulate research into the causes and improved treatment of mental illness. It should (but does not inevitably) lead to a better understanding of mental illness and hence, through education and public awareness, a reduction in stigmatisation and exclusion. Being aware – and acknowledging the high prevalence and the great burden – of mental illness is the beginning of a long process of dragging madness out of the shadows of ignorance and denial and shame.

A report – *The Global Burden of Disease: A comprehensive assessment of mortality and disability from diseases, injuries and risk factors in 1990 and projected to 2020* – was published in 1990 by the Harvard School of Public Health on behalf of the World Health Organization and the World Bank. In a summary of the findings, the writers made one observation that they described as 'startling'. The burdens of mental illnesses had been underestimated by traditional approaches that take mortality but not disability into account. While psychiatric conditions are responsible for just over one per cent of deaths, they account for almost eleven per cent of the disease burden worldwide. Of the ten leading causes of disability, five were neuropsychiatric disorders. In the projected estimates of the disease burden for 2020, depression was second only to ischaemic heart disease.

There is even greater cause for concern in that indirect psychiatric causes of mortality are not reflected in these figures. People living with serious mental illnesses have a life expectancy that is reduced by ten to twenty years. There are many reasons for this very disturbing figure but high among them are smoking and a lack of exercise and self-care in general, which are significant risk factors for premature death due to cerebrovascular and respiratory diseases.

There is no correspondence between these estimates of disease burden and resource allocation or the funding of research. The problems are compounded by a 'treatment gap' in that only about twenty-five per cent of those living with mental illnesses are estimated to receive the treatment they require. There are many probable reasons for this – including ignorance and hence stigma and rejection – but it seems that, beyond these more readily identifiable factors, there is a more mysterious and profound failure or unwillingness to grasp the grim realities of mental illness.

In many low- and middle-income countries, other factors including poverty, violence and gender inequality constitute risk factors for psychiatric morbidities. Poverty and mental illness interact in a negative cycle of misfortune. For a host of reasons, poverty significantly increases the risk of mental illness, and mental illness leads very often to poverty. Children and the elderly are particularly vulnerable. Major social and economic changes and upheavals such as urbanisation and migration undermine stable family and community support systems, and contribute further to poor outcomes.

The growing awareness reflected in these epidemiological studies of the global burden of psychiatric disorders and their enormous social and economic impact is important and potentially valuable in reprioritising resources and research funding. In most low- and middle-income countries, less than two per cent of the total health budget is allocated to mental-health services. The figures cannot, however, indicate the hardships and inestimable suffering of those struggling with mental illnesses, nor of their families and communities. The plight of the mentally ill, especially in low- and middle-income countries, is lamentable and unjust.

The high prevalence of, and the burdens owing to disability need to be confronted and acknowledged. This is an important first step in taking the necessary action to prevent and limit disability. The problem needs to be understood as a human-rights issue, rather than one arising inevitably from impairments of psychological and social functioning. Harm arises from the misperceptions of disability as irreversible, and therefore a sufficient reason for the fatalistic attitude that there is not much more that can be done other than the provision of a disability grant. Being identified as disabled too often entails the neglect of the necessary effort to foster resilience.

An alternative response would be to identify specific disabilities with the aim of doing whatever might be necessary to prevent a person's life from becoming unnecessarily restricted or thwarted. But this is not enough. It might be more helpful to regard disability not as an individual problem but more as a political issue. Social discrimination on the grounds of mental illness is a human-rights violation. It also impoverishes us all. Treating this human and complex problem as a political issue requires us to consider ways of fostering more tolerant and humane attitudes, rather than a more restricted notion of an obligation merely to rehabilitate an afflicted person back into a society that many might regard as itself being sick, fragmented and hostile. The problems are compounded by the changing nature of the world we inhabit. In an increasingly materialistic and technological culture, the potential for alienation seems all the more likely to undermine such possibly utopian fantasies. All the more effort is then required to create and maintain attitudes of acceptance and inclusion and compassion. The disability of an individual should not be allowed to shift attention away from the disabling social attitudes for which we all share a responsibility and which shape our own lives.

A mother wrote to me of her son living with schizophrenia:

> While there were times that the situation seemed to be completely hopeless, I gradually became more determined that my son's con-

> dition would improve. I refused to accept that he would need to be permanently disabled.

She described a number of interventions, including adjusting his medication, his becoming a member of a well-supervised group home and her joining a support group.

> Our lives are much better now. My son has been stable for years ... he is compliant with the medication and even grudgingly accepts that he does have an illness that requires treatment. He has started a small business that gives him the dignity of earning his own spending money and he is learning to drive. These are milestones that I really celebrate. He spends weekends with me and it is a pleasure now to be in his company. But one of the most thrilling events for me is that he has discovered how to laugh again. Not the sort of laughing that he used to do when he was obviously delusional, and which filled me with fear. Now he is able to appreciate humour and he regularly roars with laughter when he recognises the fun and joy of an experience. I know he will never be the young man that I dreamt he would be, but I have learnt to accept that nevertheless he is a sensitive, loving and considerate person and I am very proud of him.

It has been a struggle. She says she has learnt to see what has happened to both of them in a different light. In an imaginative and helpful way, she has refused to think of her son as disabled; she has retrieved a sense of pride and joy in her relationship with him. Clearly, both of them have benefited. The status conferred of disability should be a means towards helping. It should not be a trap.

17

It's all in the mind

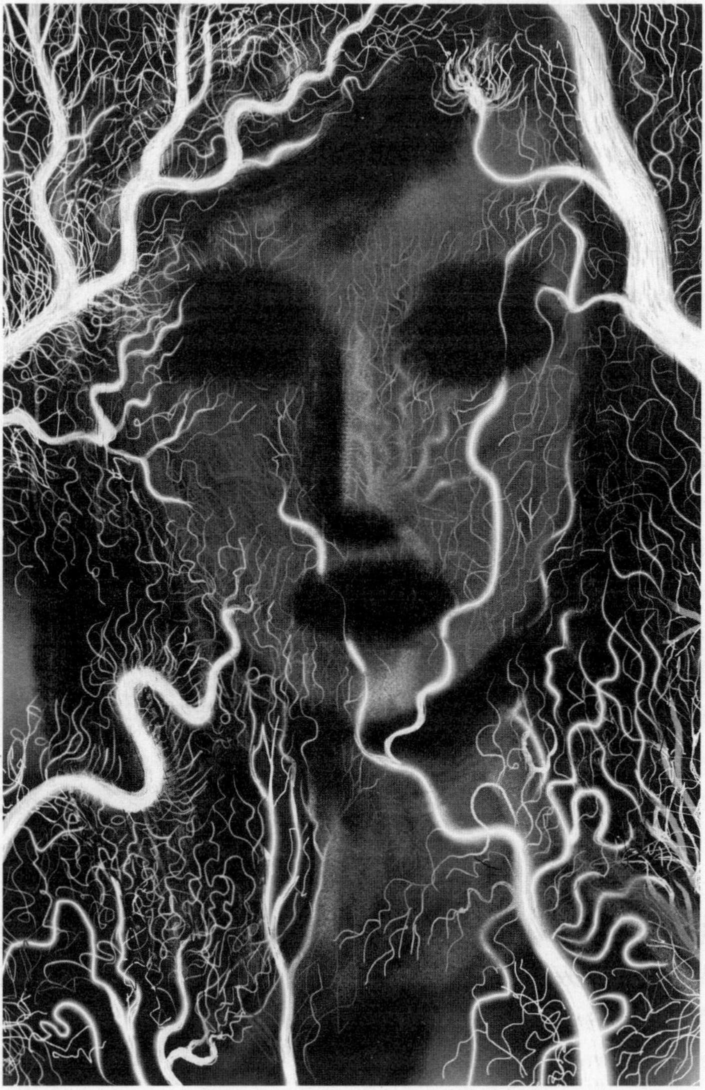

Hlaudi is screaming in one of the dormitories. The patients are terrified. The nurses are running towards him. Blood is pouring from one of his eyes. He is trying to fight off the nurses but is flailing blindly. The doctor on call is summoned urgently. Hlaudi has taken a spoon from the kitchen and has used it to try and remove his eye. The eye is badly damaged. An ambulance is called and he is taken to the general hospital where the surgeons attempt to save his eye. Too much damage has been done. The eye is surgically removed and Hlaudi returns to the ward. Why has he done this to himself? He cannot give a clear answer, other than to say he was told to do it. He had no control, he says. He was made to take out his eye. Now he is frightened and angry. He is inconsolable.

All in the mind?

Johan is a successful businessman. He is married with two children. On the surface all is well. There is nothing he tells us that can explain the depression that has descended upon him. He has become incapacitated. His colleagues at work have insisted that he take time off. They say he must sort himself out, otherwise he will be asked to leave the business he started. His wife is bewildered. She is also afraid. She tells us that a close relative committed suicide and that her husband has never been able to talk to her about it. She fears he will do the same. She has never seen him in this state. He is transformed. He stares at her and the children blankly. They reach out to touch him but he flinches. He takes no care of himself. He barely speaks. He mutters. He sighs. He does not seem to hear them.

'This is not my Johan,' the wife cries. 'This is not the father of my children. Johan, please talk to us. Tell us what is the matter with you.'

He looks away.

Is this all merely in his mind?

Marcia has lived with pain for most of her adult life. She was a lively, energetic young woman, a keen and very talented tennis player. Her ambition was to become a professional. In her final year at school she strained a ligament in her left leg and was advised to rest for a few weeks.

The pain persisted and steadily got worse. It spread to both lower limbs and then, to her great dismay, insidiously and remorselessly it engulfed her whole body. She was distraught. She tried everything. Nothing worked. The physiotherapist could not explain it. Nor could the general practitioner. Nor could a chiropractor. She became angry when a tennis partner suggested that she was exaggerating the pain. She was increasingly desperate. What was to become of her ambitions to become a professional tennis player? What was happening to her? Eventually she consulted an orthopaedic surgeon. He examined her thoroughly and did a number of investigations. He told her there was nothing wrong with her. He said: 'It's all in your mind.'

All in the mind? Not real? Was she 'putting it on' – and if so, for what purpose?

It is all in the mind, because that is where consciousness resides, but that is not what 'it's all in the mind' means. What we usually mean is that, in some deeply strange way, it is not there.

When telling me of this encounter Marcia becomes agitated. She is understandably indignant. If her pain is not real, if it is all in her mind, the explanation could only be that she is making it up, that she is malingering. The implicit allegation is that she is seeking to deceive. This is altogether too much after all the suffering she has been through. Anger and mistrust now compound her misery.

I try to explain to her, I think without much success, where the surgeon's comments come from. We are trained to think in an evidence-based, biomedical framework. A patient presents with some symptom or another. We take a history and perform an examination and request special investigations to seek objective evidence of the diagnosis to explain the symptom. We might prescribe medication not on a whim but on the basis of evidence derived from randomised, controlled clinical trials.

This is all very well, but it falls apart in the above circumstances. For Hlaudi and Johan and Marcia, there are no objective signs or special investigations to explain their suffering. To then infer that their symptoms are not real is clearly nonsense. To further infer that the distress arising from these symptoms is not real, and that the symptoms are fabricated, is offensive. It is certainly not helpful.

I see Alicia in the neurology ward. She suffers from epilepsy. She is a bright, surprisingly cheerful woman in her early twenties. She has coped relatively well with the condition that developed when she was a child. She is diligent in taking her anti-epileptic medication. She managed to complete her schooling, gaining sufficiently good grades to consider a course in advertising. She was admitted to the neurology ward because her seizures have mysteriously become more frequent in the past few months. For the first time since the diagnosis was made, the epilepsy appears to be out of control.

I am asked to see her because there is also something odd about the seizures the staff have observed. The usual stereotyped pattern is not described and the convulsions continue for much longer than normal. There is no customary shaking, but more of a wild and atypical writhing. During this time her eyes are held tightly closed. The incontinence that may accompany such generalised seizures is not observed and there is no self-injurious behaviour. The reflexes are not brisk, as usually noted during seizures. When these curious episodes end she appears to wake up suddenly, saying, 'Where am I? What happened?' More usually after a seizure patients are confused and it takes some minutes to regain full consciousness. The electroencephalograms show no indication of recent seizure activity. My colleagues are mystified. Are these real seizures? Is she faking them – and if so, why?

I tell Alicia that there is some uncertainty about the nature of her seizures. There has been a change in the pattern and frequency, and this is unusual. I ask if I can make some enquiries about what is going on in her life. She says she is struggling. She is deeply anxious about embarking on the advertising course. She does not know whether she will cope, or whether she should tell the course supervisors about her epilepsy. She believes that her boyfriend is about to leave her. He says he is scared of the seizures. She thinks he is embarrassed to be associated with somebody with epilepsy. There are tensions in her parents' marriage. She fears they are about to divorce and she blames herself for the stress her epilepsy might have put on the marriage.

Alicia is not faking these seizures, but neither are they seizures due to her epilepsy. The convulsions are not under her voluntary control. The terminology is confused. The word 'hysteria' is of the past, and derogatory. In the domain of neurology these episodes would be described as non-epileptic convulsions; in psychiatry a diagnosis of a conversion disorder would probably be made. In this respect, a symptom – very often of a neurological nature – is thought to arise not from a neurological disorder but from psychological and social stressors. The symptom is not intentionally produced and it does not preclude there being a neurological or any other disorder.

I explain this to Alicia in a way I hope will make sense to her. She does not appear to have any difficulty in accepting what I say. A referral is made for both her and her parents to see a clinical psychologist.

I am later told that things have settled down. The convulsions have subsided. She was advised to tell the course supervisors of her epilepsy and to her great relief they told her that it should not in any way prejudice her application. Her parents were able to reassure her that there was no substance to her fears that they were about to separate. The boyfriend went on his way but she told the psychologist that she did not want to be with anybody who was scared or embarrassed by her diagnosis.

Psychiatric problems have physical effects, and general medical conditions can have very serious psychiatric consequences – but these associations themselves make implicit assumptions of a mind–body dualism. The mind is inherently embodied. There is no mind outside our bodies. Conversely, the body can be without mind, as in dementia or a persistent vegetative state following a stroke or a traumatic head injury. The brainstem is intact so the person breathes, the heart beats, but at the higher cortical level there is no activity. There is no consciousness, no mind, only a profound and terrible stillness.

The most obvious and dramatic physical consequence of a psychiatric disorder is suicide. It makes no sense to consider suicide as being all in the mind. Another consequence is anorexia. Anorexia can be life-threatening. It is a deeply mysterious condition. The factors that contribute to its emergence are wide-ranging and interactive and include, importantly, social and cultural influences. That does not make anorexia any less dangerous, or all in the mind. It does seem possible that this misunderstanding or this false assumption that anorexia is somehow a psychological rather than a medical disorder contributes to the anguish and the anger that attends this condition. It might also entrench symptoms to convince sceptics of the veracity of the patient's predicament.

More commonly, psychological factors affect the way a person might cope with a medical disorder. Busisiwe is a vivacious young woman who struggles to accept a diagnosis of systemic lupus erythematosus (SLE). It is not possible that this is something she is going to have to live with, that there is no cure. It is not fair. She just wants to be normal, she says. She doesn't want to be a patient. She doesn't want to be bloated with the steroids she will need to take. She doesn't want people fussing over her, pretending not to notice her rashes.

SLE is all the more complicated because of its erratic and unpredictable course. It waxes and wanes. When the symptoms remit Busisiwe insists that it is all over. There will be no recurrence and she will no longer need to take the treatment. When the rash reappears on her face she is angry and grief-stricken. She rebels. She drops out of school. She begins to use drugs. She becomes promiscuous and she is pregnant at the age of eighteen. Her parents are distraught and helpless. What might have been manageable with difficulty has become increasingly unmanageable. Her future has become bleak.

Khalid is also eighteen and he is also angry. He struggles to accept that he has insulin-dependent diabetes. At one level he understands that without rigorous control of his blood sugars he can become gravely ill. At another level he is disbelieving. He is also defiant. He uses the insulin sporadically. He eats with disregard to sugar. His parents find him comatose in his bedroom. He is rushed to the emergency unit of the local hospital where a diagnosis is made of a diabetic ketoacidosis. He fights with the nurses. He is abusive towards the doctors. This chaotic course continues. Khalid remains deeply resentful of his illness and his adherence to treatment is sporadic. Five years after the diagnosis was first made his left foot is amputated due to an uncontrolled infection. Khalid says he is now a cripple and he is useless and his life is over. Is this all in the mind?

A very wide range of general medical conditions can present with psychiatric symptoms. For this reason every patient undergoes a physical examination on admission to the ward. The great dread is delirium. This can be subtle in that a slightly altered level of consciousness might be difficult to discern, all the more so in a young person who is psychotic and behaviourally disturbed. If missed the consequences can be dire.

Willem is a middle-aged man with schizophrenia whom I see regularly in the outpatient clinic. He is pleasant and diffident in his manner, and for some time there has been a degree of stability in his illness. When I see him he is calm and bemused by the anxieties expressed by the staff of the group home where he has lived for years. They say he was not quite himself. There is nothing else. He says he is fine. I report back to the concerned staff. No, they say, there was something wrong. They know him well and something in him has changed. I make an appointment to see him in two weeks' time. He says again that there is no problem and that the anxieties of the staff are unfounded. On this occasion, at the conclusion of the meeting and after getting up from the chair, his left foot drags as he turns to leave the room.

A CT scan shows a large tumour in the frontal cortex of his brain. The staff have been remarkably alert to a subtle shift in his behaviour and did not make the idle assumption that any symptom should be attributed to the schizophrenia. Unfortunately it was too late and Willem died six weeks later.

There are many reasons why people with severe psychiatric disorders have a reduced life expectancy. One is a bizarre assumption that having been diagnosed with a mental illness, persons become disembodied. The mind is not in some separate realm to the body. How mind emerges from matter may be a mystery but the neural correlates of consciousness are not.

This confused thinking about the mind in relation to the brain contributes to the stigma associated with mental illnesses. Being intangible and non-substantive, disorders of the mind are perceived as not sharing the gravity of bodily illnesses. It is baffling that the very faculty that makes us who we are in this casual and non-reflective way should be considered to be not quite real.

18

At least it's not going to kill you

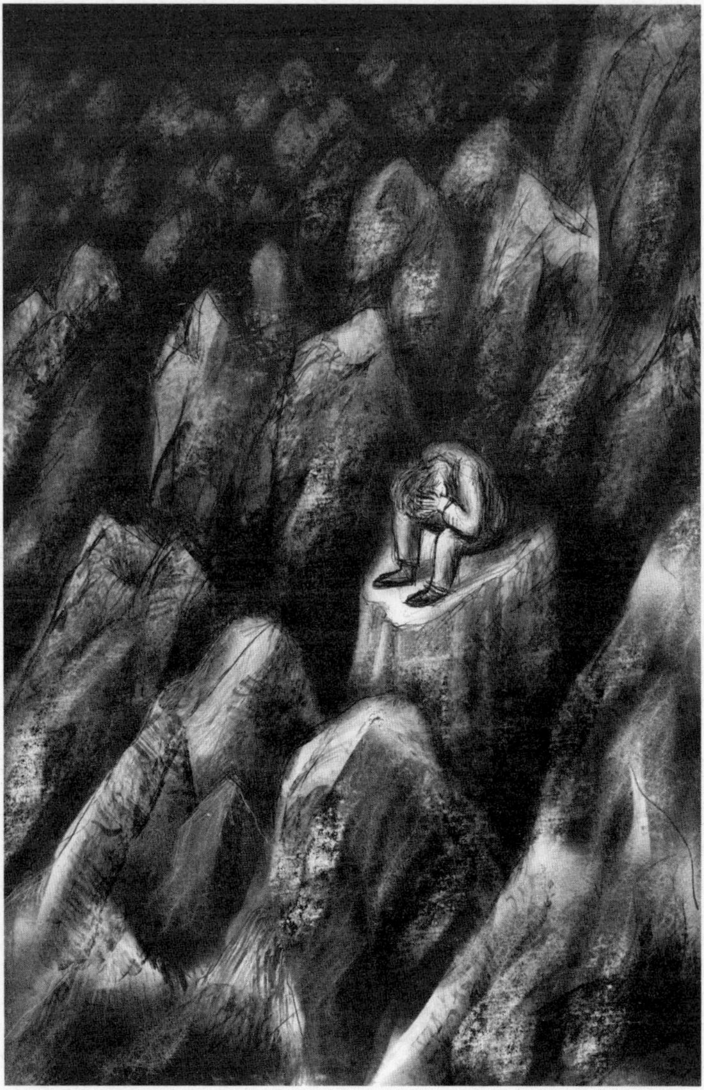

Psychiatric disorders are of less import and less deserving of medical attention because they don't kill you. This is of particular concern in low- and middle-income countries where resources are limited. Treatment of diseases with the highest mortality rates should be the first priority. Anxiety and depression might be widely prevalent, but because these disorders don't kill you they cannot warrant the consideration and the means necessary to save lives. Resource-rich first-world countries might be able to afford the luxury of increased spending for mental-health services. The rest of the world cannot.

Mortality is a crude and limited indicator of disease severity. Rheumatoid arthritis, and many other musculoskeletal problems, are causes of widespread disability and suffering, as are chronic obstructive airways diseases and a wide range of endocrine and metabolic disorders. If properly managed, these disorders don't kill you. This does not make them less serious, either as a cause of suffering or as items of economic cost.

A broader definition of disease severity is the concept of disease burden. A widely used measure is the DALY, or estimate of disability-adjusted life years. This represents healthy years lost due to disease. It incorporates both mortality and disability, and is an estimate of the difference between the current health status and an imagined state of health in which a person might live without disease or disability to old age. The burden is measured in both medical and economic terms. The medical burden is a measure of morbidity and mortality, morbidity indicating the number of those who are unwell or disabled and mortality the number of people in a population who die prematurely as a result of a specific disease or disability.

The economic burden is direct, involving for example costs of providing medical services, and indirect, involving for example losses to the economy owing to lost productivity. The DALY itself is a limited measure. It does not reflect pain and suffering, and makes certain assumptions regarding values or the quality of life. It is uncertain whether a premature death is preferable to a life prolonged in suffering. The burden of disease also focuses on the negative and does not address the important factors that promote wellness and protect against disease and disability.

According to a series of World Health Organization studies the leading cause of disease burden measured in terms of DALY are cardiovascular disorders. The second leading cause estimated for 2020 is depression. Mortality due to heart disease might be decreasing owing to improved diagnosis and treatment but disability would then be increasing. There is no hard distinction between what kills you or disables you or causes you suffering.

It does not make any sense that mental illnesses are less important than general medical conditions because they don't kill you, even in terms of the limited but objective measures of the burden of disease. This notion is nevertheless prevalent, especially in areas where conflicts inevitably arise over the appropriate allocation of limited resources and where these conflicts are driven by ignorance or ill-founded assumptions about the nature of mental illness.

Putting aside these concerns, psychiatric disorders are important causes of mortality, particularly in younger people. Suicide is the second most common cause of death in people aged fifteen to twenty-nine. This is a global figure. The statistics will always be imprecise, but for each person who kills themselves it is estimated that five attempt to do so. The great majority of suicides occur in low- or middle-income countries. This is a shameful indicator of the ignorance and hence lack of care provided to those who suffer from mental illnesses.

More common are the more subtle and complicated ways in which mental illnesses contribute to disability and reduced life expectancy. Psychiatric disorders do kill, directly and most dramatically through suicide, but more often indirectly, owing to the very nature of mental illness.

I am especially affected by Timothy's story because we were the same age and were at school together. He was extremely bright and matriculated with distinction. After finishing school we drifted apart. He embarked on a degree in architecture and I studied English and philosophy before medicine. It was to my great dismay that many years later we met again, with him now as my patient.

It was unclear, as it often is, how it all began. There was no obvious family history, but again this is often the case. A father or mother might disappear or die prematurely, and it is not known whether they or an uncle or aunt or grandparent might have suffered from some form of mental illness. Often shame obscures the truth. Timothy used drugs during his undergraduate years, but of course this was not uncommon and his use was not extreme. The drugs would have been described as 'soft', which is a meaningless term. Timothy was just doing what many other young people were doing at the time, but for him the consequences were disastrous.

He started to struggle academically, which was mystifying to his parents. There was no doubt that he was intellectually gifted but he seemed increasingly incapable of focusing his attention. This was attributed to the drugs – or perhaps, it was rather desperately argued, he was too bright and bored by the course. Things got steadily worse and he failed his third-year examinations. He refused to return to university the following year.

At about this time, he married and started a family. It was expected that this was just a difficult phase, and hoped that maybe the stability of a family might aid the process of regaining control of his life. This was not to be. He became remote from his family. His wife said he was not a father to his children. He declared himself to be an artist but his drawings became increasingly disorganised and inept. Slowly and agonisingly it became apparent to his family that he was ill.

He then abandoned his wife and his young children. He disappeared, and then re-emerged insisting that he was a rock star. He took to the streets, hammering at a broken guitar and singing raucously and without restraint or skill. He was unkempt. He began to jabber incoherently.

Eventually his appalled estranged wife made an application for him to be assessed, and after some time he was admitted to our unit and I became his doctor.

Timothy greets me amicably; it seems he wishes to pretend that it is just a chance meeting of two old school friends. There is no problem, he says. It is all just a misunderstanding, perhaps a failure on the part of his family to recognise his genius. He is experimenting, he tells me, but he does rather begrudgingly acknowledge that he might have gone too far. He is affronted to find himself in a psychiatric hospital. It is ridiculous, he insists, that he should be punished for bravely going where no other more timid souls would venture.

To my dismay, but to the amused delight of the other patients and the nurses, he starts to sing with abandon to prove the point that he is exceptionally talented. It is not a success. I register with sadness the puzzlement he shows when it dawns upon him that others do not share his exalted opinion of his singing ability. He becomes crestfallen. He is confused. Perhaps something is wrong. Perhaps he is ill in some strange way and needs some form of help. He is broken.

Begrudgingly he accepts the need for medication. Things calm down for a while. He puts aside his battered guitar, resigning himself to the reality that he is not a rock star. After a few weeks we discharge him from the unit. When I see him in the outpatient clinic he is subdued and depressed. What does his life now hold for him without the glorious status of being a star? His movements are slow and lethargic. The tone of his speech is flat. He is making an effort, he says, but he indicates that he feels his life is empty.

His wife and children have finally left him. The children now refuse to have any contact with him. They tell me that they have to get on with their lives and that he has wrought too much havoc and that they cannot imagine that any form of reconciliation is ever going to be possible. His wife makes occasional contact with him but there is no longer any intimacy between them. She is understandably angry and says she has tried but that she no longer believes that there was anything that she could do to help him.

He is spending most of his time listlessly with the other residents of the group home. They do not do very much. They smoke. They watch television and rarely leave the home. Timothy grows bored and restless. It is inevitable that this wan life should become to him an intolerable compromise and that he should again seek the raptures of stardom.

So back he comes, beating furiously on the guitar that he has retrieved, wailing and shouting and shrieking in some mad belief that his performance is anything other than a discordant din. After yet another admission he resigns himself to the drab realities of a life that he begins to believe has been stricken by his illness.

When we meet again in the outpatient clinic he looks unhealthy. He is overweight and breathes with difficulty. He is smoking far too much and does no exercise. He is not looking after himself. He says he doesn't care; smoking is one of the few meagre pleasures in his life.

His difficulties are compounded by the side-effects of the medications he has reluctantly come to accept he needs. Over the years recourse has been taken to the use of increasingly powerful agents to bring him out of his psychotic states, and these medications have had inevitably severe and problematic effects on his physical well-being. Although only taken at night one agent is powerfully sedating. Other important side-effects are weight gain and blood lipid or fat disorders. Not exercising, smoking excessively and doing very little with regard to basic health care, our patients are at grave risk of a host of medical issues, including respiratory problems and cardiovascular events, or heart attacks, which are largely responsible for the reduced life expectancy of people living with schizophrenia.

Months later Timothy is struggling to breathe. He tells me that he has been diagnosed with chronic obstructive airways disease. He becomes even more sedentary. His rock star days are over – now it is an endeavour just to keep going. Showing great determination and strength of character, which is all the more remarkable in his depleted circumstances, he resolves to stop smoking. It is all too late. His breathlessness grows worse. When I see him again he seems much older than his years. It baffles and dismays me that we are the same age, and it seems profoundly unjust that this physical deterioration has been so unfairly wrought upon him by a mental illness for which he could hold no responsibility.

On the next occasion he shuffles into the interview room on crutches. His pallor is grey. He can barely speak. He says he has been diagnosed with advanced lung cancer. A decision has been made to treat him with radiotherapy. He shrugs; to my distress I form the impression that he has given up.

Weeks later the manager of the group home asks me to visit him in the general hospital where he is being treated for the cancer. He is bedridden but speaks to me warmly and coherently. He says he is unable to move and that this is a mystery to the physicians who are treating him. There is no explanation on medical grounds for why he is unable to rise from his bed. He does not appear to be depressed. He is calmer and seems to be more at peace with himself and his circumstances than I have observed for years. He dies days later.

Timothy's far too early demise was a consequence of the schizophrenia from which he suffered for most of his life. The illness did not kill him directly, but in many interacting and indirect ways, including his self-injurious behaviour, the effects of medication, a lack of basic self-care and, finally and most importantly, the loss I think of the will to live.

It is nonsense to say that at least mental illness doesn't kill you, because it can and it does, and also because mortality is no measure of the worth and value of life.

19

The cliché of the madness of the world

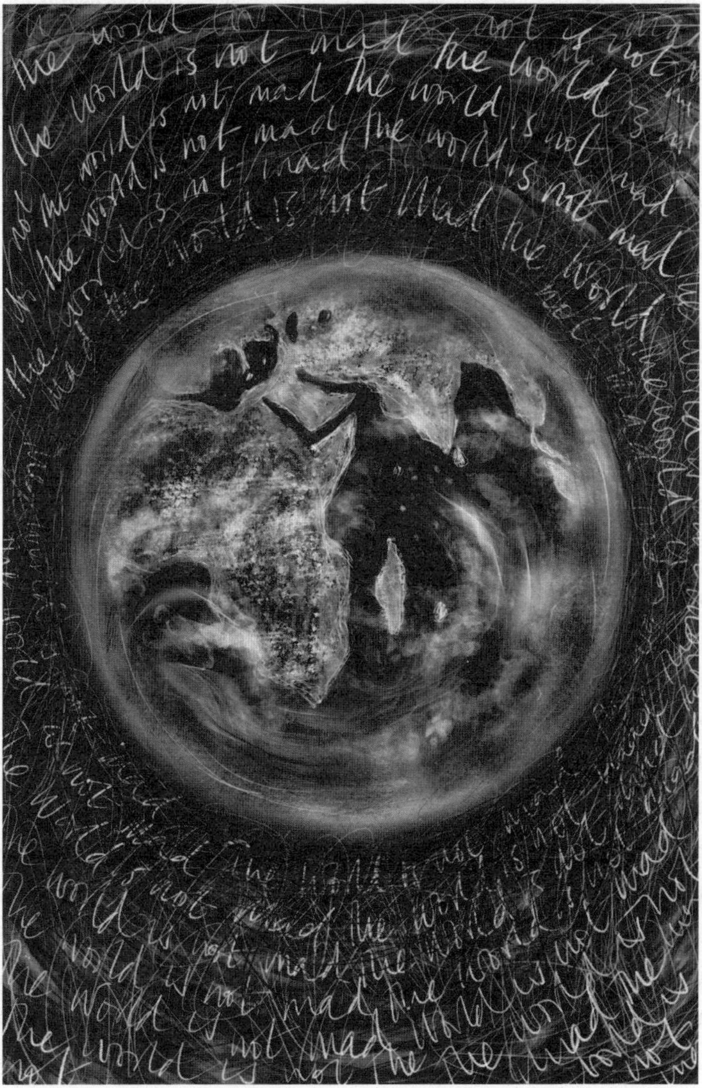

The world is not mad. That the world is mad is a ridiculous proposition, but it is said again and again. Presumably the statement is intended to convey a deep insight into the strangeness and the irrationality of the world in which we live, but the world is not a person and strangeness and irrationality do not equate to madness. It is a glib and fatuous contention and for many of those who suffer from serious mental illness it might be considered a dismissive cliché.

Mary has lived with schizophrenia for most of her life and so has her mother. They both come to see me in the outpatient clinic but the mother is managed in the private sector. She accompanies her daughter because the daughter becomes anxious and muddled when she is on her own. The mother does not have confidence that her daughter will tell me the truth about what is happening to her. To some extent, she is right. Mary is eager to please. Although she is in her late thirties her manner is childlike. She wishes to reassure me that all is going well and that she is coping and making a great effort not to allow things to get her down.

The mother seems tired and exasperated. 'Tell him,' she says. 'Tell him what happened yesterday.' Mary becomes anxious and tearful. I don't think she wants to tell me what happened yesterday. Maybe she is embarrassed. Maybe it has not gone away, whatever it might have been. The mother insists. She is impatient. She is sick of all this, she tells me. She is getting older. Who is going to look after Mary when she is no longer capable? And anyway, she tells me, she herself is not well and in no position to help Mary when she suffers these psychotic episodes. She has no support. Both Mary's siblings have long since left home, one to a city up north and the other to the UK. It seems very probable that they both have fled from a situation that they found suffocating and that the only way they felt they could survive was to separate themselves physically from their troubled mother and sister.

Mary clearly does not want to discuss the events of the previous day, but the mother says, 'How is the doctor supposed to help you if you don't tell him? You can't go on pretending that everything is all right. You are not well.' Mary is sobbing now. The mother turns away. This has happened too often. She does not know what to do. Mary will not allow her to leave the room. She needs her mother and her mother cannot help.

'It's terrible,' she says. It is Albert, one of the residents, or it could be Julian or Thabo or Yusuf or Jacob. Whoever it is on this occasion is tormenting her. 'He is trying to hurt me. I know he is. I can see it by the way he is looking at me at the breakfast table, by the way he is holding his knife. He is putting terrible thoughts into my mind. He wants to hurt me. Why is he doing this to me? I have done nothing to him. I thought he was my friend, but now I can see he hates me. He wants to destroy me. It is so unfair. It's terrible. I want to die.'

Now the mother is in tears. 'It's nonsense,' she says. 'It's all in your mind. It is just not true. You are unwell. It's just your imagination. Nobody wants to hurt you. Everybody likes you. Everybody is trying to help you.'

When Mary has eventually left to collect her medication, the mother says that on this occasion Mary started to scream uncontrollably and had to be removed from the breakfast room. This caused great distress among the other residents. The manageress has told Mary's mother that she does not think the situation can continue. It is not fair to the other residents. Unless something is done – and presumably this means that unless her psychiatrist is able to sort out her medication – she very sadly will have to consider asking Mary to leave.

'What am I to do, Doctor? She can't come back to stay with me. I am not well myself. I am not strong, and anyway it's not safe. I know it. It's the neighbours. They are pumping poison through the ceiling of my flat. They are trying to get me out. Nobody will believe me but it's true. Mary cannot come to stay with me. I won't be able to cope. I will get sick again. Please, Doctor, you have to help us.'

This is not the madness of the world. I cannot say to this family, 'Oh, this is just the way things are. You just need to resign yourselves. The world is mad anyway. There is nothing exceptional in your predicament.' Perhaps I might justify such idiotic contentions if I thought it might be therapeutic to change anguish into rage but I think that is fanciful.

One implication of this cliché is that it trivialises mental illness and in this way fails to acknowledge or blithely dismisses the suffering of patients and their families. Another imputation, and I am not sure if this is made with fully conscious intent, is that there really is no such thing as mental illness. If the world is mad anyway, however ludicrous the notion might be, there is no validity to the phenomenon of mental illness – or, in a postmodern context, it is relative to the point of meaninglessness.

Such careless platitudes are not without consequence and do harm. It is difficult for me in the encounter with Mary and her mother to convey to them with confidence that I will be able to help, but mouthing cruel banalities could certainly not be construed as a constructive intervention.

There is a tension between acknowledging the grim reality and the suffering associated with mental illness and the need to be helpful and to be hopeful. Perhaps it is yet another cliché to describe clinical practice as an art, but this does to some extent indicate the limits of the biomedical framework and the need to attend to the uniqueness of each presentation. The scientific perspective is both necessary and helpful, but in this encounter there are no fundamental and objectively verifiable strategies that can guide me in how to respond to this mother's plea. It does require some form of creative balance, being both hopeful and realistic, and there is no knowing whether we get it right – or how often, if at all, or what being right might be.

These difficulties cannot distract those involved from addressing the complex nature of mental illness and the problem of delineating its boundaries, but the dismissal of boundaries altogether in the flippant assertion that the world is mad makes no useful or serious contribution.

A linked and equally exasperating cliché that I have had to contend with far too often is the observation that we are all mad. This is delivered as a profound insight, frequently over a glass of wine or on some social occasion where to take issue would cast one as being earnest and boring. Being mad in this sense would appear to be free, to be one's true self, unfettered by social convention, to joyfully discard the constraints of whatever might quite arbitrarily be considered normal.

It is again unclear whether the consequences of this have been thoughtfully considered. Perhaps part of my irritation is due to the implication that if we are all mad the notion of mental illness has no validity, and the profession of psychiatry is therefore fraudulent. In this regard psychiatrists are not doctors, seeking to alleviate distress and restore a degree of function in those diagnosed with mental illness, but social police, seeking to maintain order – and, taking it further, punishing those who stray with incarceration and stupefying medications. Psychiatrists are agents of the state, tasked with maintaining the status quo. Healing, according to this position, is merely bringing the wayward back into the fold. It is fundamentally coercive. People with political opinions that are regarded as a threat to the security of the state, or that are simply awkward, have been – and no doubt continue to be – considered mentally ill in many parts of the world and excluded in different ways from society. This is an egregious and cynical abuse of psychiatry.

I do not doubt that there are malpractices in psychiatry and in general medicine, and I do not doubt that psychiatry in particular is prone to such malpractices. There are many reasons for this, among which are the absence of any objective signs of mental illness and, related to this, the shifting and extending boundaries of what might be considered to constitute mental illness.

Mrs Khumalo seems irritable and impatient. We are gathered in a ward round and she has been describing to us the ordeal of getting her son Manto into hospital. A group of medical students are attending. I am required in the interests of the discipline of psychiatry to ask questions that might lead us to a diagnosis. Following the conventions of clinical medicine, this is necessarily a systematic and ordered process. It is not merely that an impression is gained, or that a few vague and arbitrary questions throw up a random diagnosis. These diagnoses have significant consequences. They might provide access to a disability grant but they can also be stigmatising. A psychiatric diagnosis is also notorious in that it sticks to one: a diagnosis of tuberculosis for example might become something of the past; a diagnosis of schizophrenia much less so.

The questions are dutifully asked and it becomes clear from the history Mrs Khumalo provides that her son is probably suffering from schizophrenia.

There are a host of misconceptions attached to this label, so I feel obliged to confer this probable diagnosis with caution. Mrs Khumalo does not appear to be very interested. Schizophrenia, *ukuthwasa*, *amafufunyana*, *ukuthakathwa*, what does it matter, she seems to suggest. The terms are irrelevant. Her son is sick. He has gone mad. It is our duty to make him better.

The questions we ask, the labels we use and the diagnoses we propose are of much lesser import than the urgency of fixing the problem and getting her son home. She appears to be unimpressed by our attempts to be cautious and it seems likely to me that she interprets our tentativeness as a lack of certainty. Mrs Khumalo understandably wants certainty – not about any diagnosis that we might make, but that this nightmare will soon be something of the past and her son will be restored to her.

The world is not mad. Neither cruelty, injustice and inhumanity, nor mere eccentricity of behaviour, nor the refusal to conform to social convention are symptoms of mental illness. To regard these familiar characteristics of human behaviour as such is demeaning to those who suffer from mental illness.

I am not sure what might or should be the most appropriate language. 'Madness' is problematic. 'Mental illness' confines a wide and complex range of symptoms and signs of distress to a medical subspeciality. Underpinning whichever terms we use is the need to acknowledge pain and suffering, and not to dismiss these human experiences with clichés and platitudes.

20

Madness is not a metaphor

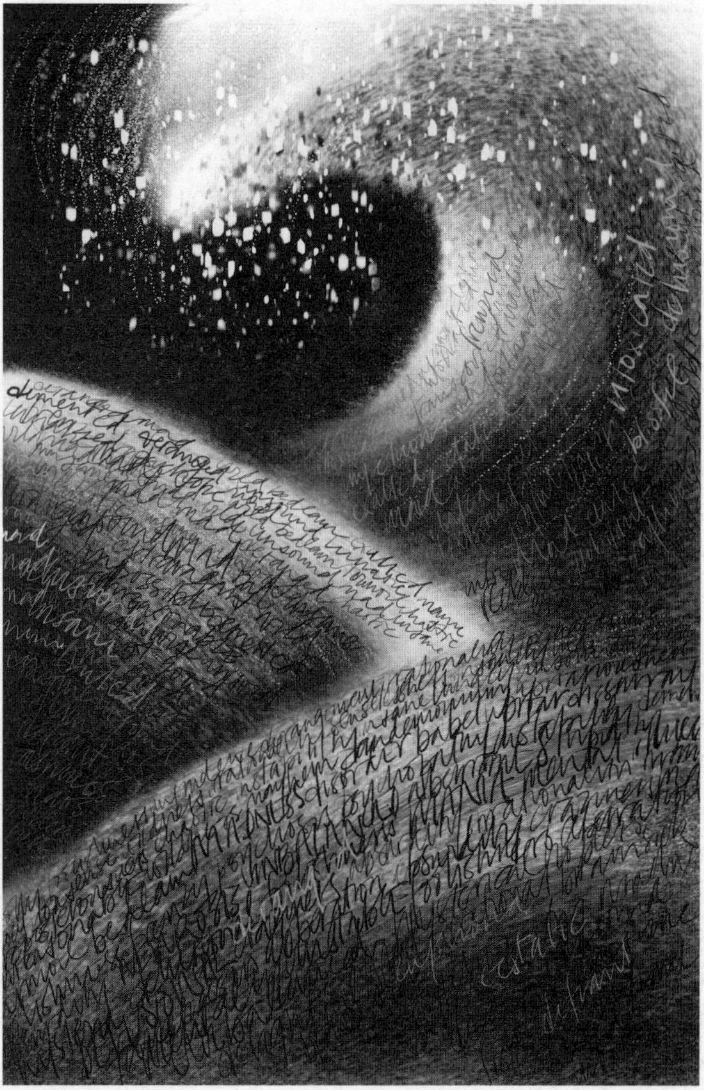

You are mad. You are sick, you are exceptional, you are very brave or stupid. I am mad. I am angry, I am intensely moved, I have been pushed beyond the limits of my endurance. It is mad. It is wonderful, it is extreme, it is profoundly ill-judged. Mad is bad. It is a mad option. In Afrikaans, the colloquial term is '*mal*'. In French, '*mal*' means 'bad'. It is good. It is maddeningly beautiful. I was so mad about her that I was mad with anger and mad with sadness when she turned against me. She was mad to refuse everything that I had to offer her. Mad is fantastic and absurd and nonsensical. A welter of metaphorical associations distorts ideas about mental illness.

Martin is sitting opposite me in one of the outpatient clinic rooms. He is earnest, determined that I should understand. 'I am not mad, Doctor. It's true.' He tells me that he is under attack. His assailants are firing bolts of electricity at him, causing him great pain and emotional distress. It is a profound injustice, he says. He has done nothing to deserve this terrible assault on his body. 'It's not fair, Doctor. It's not right. They just keep on at me. There is nothing I can do.' He is insistent that I believe him, that I accept that what is happening to him is real and not a part of his illness. Nor should I think that the excruciatingly painful bolts are figurative in any way. 'It's really happening,' he says again and again. 'It's not what you think. I'm not delusional. It's real. You must believe me.'

I am not to think that what he is experiencing is 'as if' he is being attacked. It is not 'as if' anything. It is not a metaphor. He becomes agitated, I think, by his impression that I am seeking to interpret his experience as a mere symptom of something else, an illness. He is driven by a determination that the reality of what is happening to him should be acknowledged. This need seems of greater importance to him than that the attacks should stop. Interpreting his anguish as delusional and treating it as such would be a repudiation for him of something personally meaningful. Being believed is the overriding priority.

This need I think is not sufficiently recognised in standard clinical practice and there are problematic consequences. A patient confiding these deeply strange experiences would likely feel disbelieved and therefore dismissed as mad or delusional. Any hope of developing a trusting therapeutic relationship is then undermined. This in itself might seem a rather abstract or romantic concept that is of little practical import. A therapeutic alliance ought to be integral to an aspirational standard of best clinical practice. In the grim and time-constrained routines of a busy and chaotic admission unit such an alliance is nevertheless considered unrealistic. This is wrong. Non-adherence to treatment leads to poor outcomes and early relapse and readmission rates. Believing that you are believed lays a foundation of trust that increases the likelihood of adherence to treatment – but also something beyond that, something less measurable: that you are not irredeemably other, that you are acknowledged, not invalidated.

The capacity for abstraction might itself seem a nebulous quality. It is perhaps difficult to think of it as a fundamental strategy for survival, as being essential to coping in the quotidian world. A failure of abstracting ability – in association with a constellation of other vaguely defined functions including goal formation, sequencing and problem-solving – forms part of the neurocognitive domain of deficits in schizophrenia. These contribute significantly to the disability of the disorder and to poor prognoses, and remain relatively resistant to treatment.

These impairments are not specific to schizophrenia and are encountered in other severe psychiatric disorders such as the dementias. Carers might be familiar with the confusion and wearying exasperation of an elderly family member because of sequencing problems, failing to put on his socks before his shoes, or being unable to perform the most basic and comforting tasks such as making a cup of tea, of not buttering the bread before putting it in the toaster. The relatively complex cognitive faculties underlying these apparently simple tasks are taken for granted until things fall apart, until one becomes incapacitated – perhaps more obviously in states of dementia and more insidiously in schizophrenia. The part of the brain subserving this abstracting function is known as the dorsolateral prefrontal cortex, a term that is, of course, of utter irrelevance to Martin and the exhausted carers of their demented family members.

Treating madness as a metaphor burdens Martin in different ways. What is happening to him is denied. It is a symptom of an illness that means what is happening is not really happening. It is enough to make you mad, or certainly angry. This is further complicated by the notion that this illness is not an illness at all. It is a metaphor. The metaphor itself is confused by a plethora of contradictory meanings. It is extreme, exceptional. It is evil. It is calamitous.

Martin tells me, 'I try to find a word, a barrier or protection … to rid myself of these connections induced in my body … I am bombarded by too many people, too many psychic forces … the outside world, my enemies invade my private world … it's terrible … so many nights I have been under attack.'

There is no metaphorical space in these utterances, no protective distance. He is bombarded. He is invaded. It is terrifying because it is immediate, vivid. It is so intensely real to him that he seeks to protect himself. He does not have the space or the capacity to console himself that this is not really happening to him, that it is just a terrible dream or that it is confined to his imagination. Intriguingly, his defensive strategy is language. He tries to find a word, a symbol, to create some distance, a barrier for himself against the invasion.

On the more severe end of the schizophrenia spectrum patients become mute. I have never encountered Martin in such a state of stupor but I remember Petrus clearly. He had been admitted to the unit as a matter of urgency, having withdrawn into a silent psychotic world during the preceding week. He had stopped eating and then, to the great distress of his family, he had stopped taking any fluids. They knew that if this persisted it could become a medical emergency. Perhaps most unnerving was the absence of any visible sign of distress. He was completely and profoundly unresponsive. He gazed through me. In his world I was not there. I don't think that, at that time for him, there was an external world. He had become engulfed by it. Martin had at least found some precarious protection, some distance in using the words to articulate his experience. Petrus had sunk beyond this. He was lost to us. He sat completely still in his chair, seemingly unperturbed by the dismay of those around him, remote, catatonic, utterly confounded by his internal turmoil.

'When I'm sick the machine comes on … there is no barrier … I was too much into this thing to question it … it would drive me completely insane … it's a man's worst nightmare, this remote brain control … there's no escaping it …' This is Xolani after emerging from a catatonic state that was similar in many ways to Petrus's. Like Martin, he has sought some form of barrier, but as the psychosis develops there is no escape. Like Petrus, he is too much into it to question it, to even find a language to articulate it. In these depths it is just terrifyingly happening. There are no metaphorical spaces to provide some refuge. There is no alternative reality. The wretched machine controls everything. Its pervasive force overwhelms his defences. It is a nightmare but it is not a nightmare. It is really happening. As he emerges he finds some space. He needs a metaphorical explanation for the experience he has been through. He wants me to understand. There is no pattern, nothing that he can latch onto, no life raft in the cruel sea. He infers, I think, that the remote brain control is an immersive experience, that all senses are overwhelmed and that he is drowning. He is describing to me very probably the experience in which Petrus seemed to be so hopelessly trapped.

You make me mad. It is a mad world. We use these metaphors to emphasise or expand on what we wish to convey. It is inevitable, but metaphor diminishes madness.

21

The romance of madness

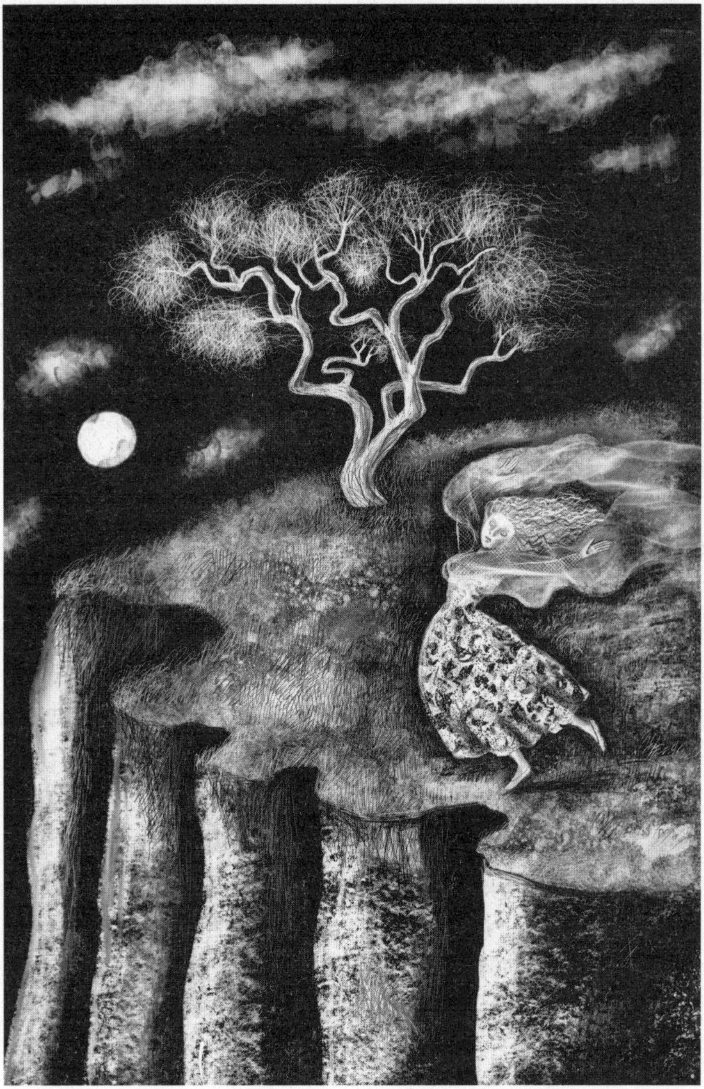

Madness is freedom. Madness is liberating. To be creative you need a little madness. Normality is confining. It is boring. It is grey. It is insipid. To impose normality is to deprive people of their right to be how they choose to be. It is to shackle them to convention. It is what the men in white coats seek to do, brandishing their syringes filled with sedating drugs. Psychiatry is inherently oppressive. Doctors and nurses work in collaboration with pharmaceutical companies and with the state to impose conformity, induce passivity and profit from what they call mental illness but what is, in reality, a heroic defiance of mediocrity.

There is an understandable need or wish to romanticise madness. Doing so would provide some comfort but it would be false. I can think of no patient who has in any way believed his or her madness to be either liberating or creative.

It is conceivable that the disinhibition, increased energy and divergent ways of thinking might dispose one to a degree of creativity, but those are not defining features of madness. There is certainly no evidence that mental illness is a requisite for creative genius and the vast majority of those who show exceptional abilities have no history of madness – just as the vast majority of those who suffer from various forms of mental illness show no signs of a special creativity. It might be argued that there is a correlation between creativity and mild and some moderate forms of mental illness but this does not apply to the psychoses. Perhaps the most obvious association is with mania. Mania fills you with energy. It vitalises you. It makes everything possible, but it does not.

Gavin only comes to see me in the outpatient clinic when he is in trouble, which is often. He is a charming, handsome man, but on this occasion he seems tired and depressed and his appearance is dishevelled. He is in pain. He hobbles awkwardly into the room on crutches. He has fractured both ankles, doing something he says was 'mad'. He had fallen from a window ledge, trying to get into a girlfriend's apartment. He says it is a crazy thing to have attempted, but that he was manic and believed that it was possible. He has been a fool, he says, and now he feels humiliated.

As has happened on so many occasions, he had stopped the mood-stabilising medications I have prescribed. He believes he does not need them. He believes they take something away from him and says, as he has said so many times, that he believes he can control his mania. I wish he could; it is ruining his life. He has been able somehow to bounce back from the damaging consequences of his manic escapades. He has laughed at the craziness of it. He construes his recklessness as exuberance but now he says he is getting tired and feeling older. It is no longer exciting. He has lost too much. His wife has left him, angry and exasperated by what she regards as his irresponsible and feckless behaviour. His children do not want to see him. They say they are teased at school because their father is mad. He has lost his job as an advertising executive. What he regarded as brilliant initiatives were dismissed by his colleagues as outlandish, and his manner towards them became increasingly hostile and contemptuous until he was asked to leave. Now his girlfriend has told him that she no longer wants to see him. What she initially considered to be high spirits she now regards as 'sick and stupid'. He tries to smile but he is dejected and forlorn. He may have been able to romanticise his manic episodes in the past, but now it is impossible and he regards his illness as a curse.

Felix has been admitted following an urgent application made by his father. He is a very large man and he is in a rage. It was one of the few occasions that I became aware that the nurses were intimidated by a patient. He is belligerent and volatile. He is also highly intelligent and entitled, making constant demands and threatening the nursing staff and the other patients with violence.

His father had contacted me a few days earlier. He was in tears. His son had assaulted him. An argument had started over a business decision. The son was a partner in the family's very successful estate agency. The son was clearly manic, and had informed his father of a proposal that the father believed would be financially ruinous. The father had told his son that he thought it was a very bad decision and that his judgement was impaired because he was ill. This had provoked the son to assault his elderly father, leading to his involuntary admission to the hospital. His fury was fuelled by his refusal to acknowledge that anything was the matter with him. It was his father who was stupid, preventing him from making a vast fortune. Everybody was stupid. Nobody understood how brilliant and rich and powerful he was. He did not belong in a hospital. We were holding him unlawfully. He would sue the health department. He would sue us all. He had very important friends in very high places and he would soon get out of hospital and do what he had to do and we would all be in a lot of trouble. This ranting went on for hours and exhausted everybody. His mania expressed itself in an arrogance that made it difficult to sympathise with him. It was difficult not to be affected by the contempt and disdain he showed us.

Felix has now sunk into a deep depression. He is listless. He is abject. He cannot work. He cannot make decisions and the business is in crisis. He has lost all motivation. He is a talented musician; in the past playing the piano was a source of great pleasure for him. Now this is inconceivable. What is the point? Nothing is going to help. There is no romance in this predicament, nor has there ever been.

There is a long and familiar list of writers and poets who have suffered from depression, with its attendant maladies of alcohol abuse and suicide. In this association there seems to be an assumption of causality, the direction of which is unclear. Is one driven into a state of depression by being more aware of the true nature of the world, and feeling a need to articulate this in some creative form, or does being depressed make us more creative, as if that is some sort of compensation or could change things? I think the association between creativity and madness is for the most part romantic. There might be some link between creativity and being of an unquiet and troubled mind, but that is not madness.

One of the most incapacitating features of a severe depression is a loss of energy and volition. You can do nothing. You want to do nothing. You are in a state of paralysis. There is no light and no shade. There is no colour. You are deprived of the very elements that are necessary to engage in any form of creative activity. Not only do you not have the energy, but you don't see any purpose in re-imagining or reconfiguring the world to make it a more interesting or a better place. It is all futile and hopeless. Alcohol might seem to provide some way of coping with this, but after a transitory and illusory lifting of the spirits it only entrenches the emptiness and the helplessness. This is not conducive to creativity.

It is possible that in states of recovery one might be motivated to try to make some sense of the experience of depression in poetry or music or in any other art form. I struggle to recall any such creative response, but then of course my involvement is partial. I don't get to see the bright side. More often there is an understandable reluctance to return to that darkness.

Finding any kind of romance in schizophrenia is even more improbable. It might be imagined that seeing things in such a different, albeit distorted, way might dispose one to creativity. Again, in my experience – for the most part limited to psychotic disorders – it does not. It disposes one to fear and avoidance.

The association of madness and creativity throughout history seems to be embedded in the popular imagination. Woolf, Plath, Hemingway, Schumann and Van Gogh are usually included in a familiar list, but there is no reason to believe that the association in these individuals and many others works in the same way. Their madness, and I doubt whether that is the right way to describe their troubled states of mind, cannot be assumed to be shared. In all probability Van Gogh would have used or suppressed his troubled spirits to make his art in quite a different way from Hemingway or Woolf. It is merely a loose association. In this respect madness seems to be more equivalent with being exceptional, or highly original, or at least not normal. These are positive attributes, not madness.

Madness does not enhance creativity. It is more likely to destroy it. It would be nice to think otherwise, it might provide at least some consolation, but in madness there is no romance.

22

Madness and the theatre

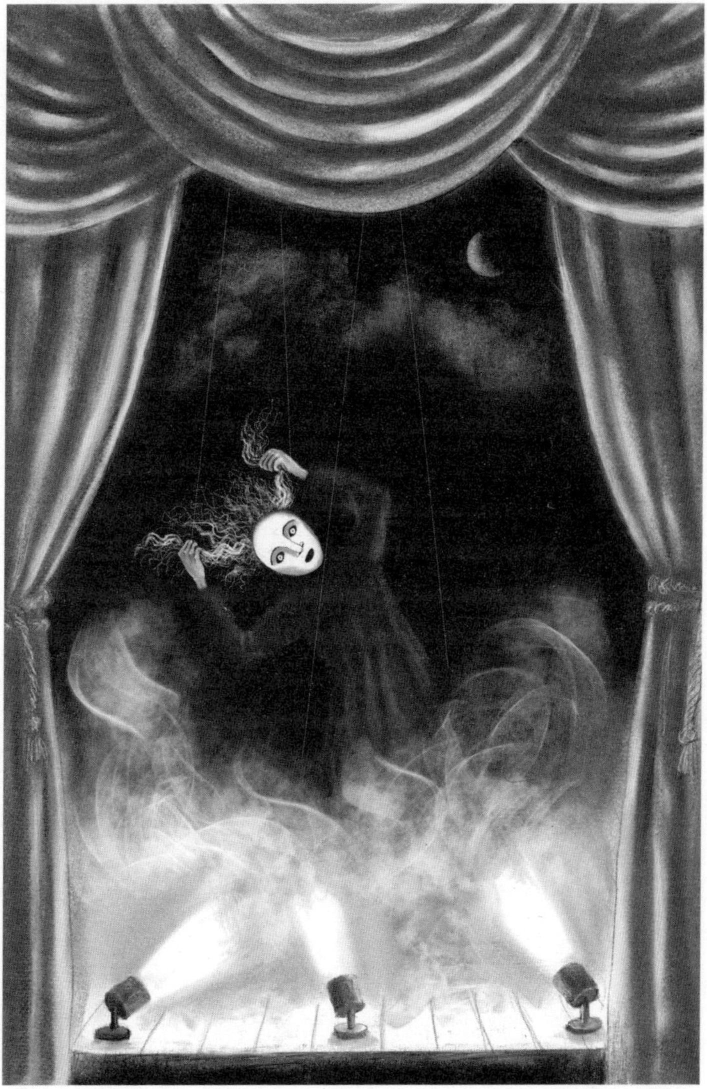

A friend who is a lecturer in theatre studies at the university asked me to talk to her students. They were planning to put on a play that involved madness, and she told me that she wanted to do this in a way that was authentic and respectful. I was impressed and agreed very willingly to meet with the students to give them at least some idea of the reality of serious mental illness. I had become exasperated by the banal and offensive stereotypes of madness so frequently and carelessly portrayed in theatre and film.

We met in one of the rehearsal rooms on campus. The students were eager and thoughtful and asked interesting and intelligent questions. I told them about my work in the admission unit of the hospital and attempted to demonstrate some of the core features of psychosis – more specifically, schizophrenia.

I remember being quite pleased with my performance of a formal thought disorder. This is probably the most difficult symptom to imitate. It is nonsense to think that patients can with ease pretend to be mad. I remember only one occasion on which a patient sought to deceive us. He was unable to sustain it for longer than twenty-four hours, and the context of his admission made it clear that he was malingering. The patients are under more or less constant surveillance. It is not possible to sustain the simulation of psychotic symptoms – in particular a formal thought disorder – for an extended period of time. I have never witnessed a remotely plausible portrayal of a formal thought disorder in any play or film.

I performed thought blocking and derailments and loosening of associations and I naïvely thought that I might have been effective in persuading the students of the need to be careful and avoid the pitfalls of melodrama and sensationalism. I was invited to the opening night. I looked forward to the performance and in particular how the lead actress playing the part of the mad young woman would portray the symptoms of psychosis that I thought we had carefully considered. On the night there was an excited atmosphere of anticipation. The director had a reputation for daring and experimental theatre work. I was unfortunately seated in the front row. The light dimmed and there was darkness and then a loud shriek and a crash and the young woman staggered onto the stage. She was completely naked and covered in faeces. She pulled her hair. She rubbed herself. She stormed about, yelling and moaning. I suppose it could be said that it was a powerful performance. It had nothing to do with schizophrenia.

I have only once encountered a naked patient covered in his own faeces. This was Francois, a portly, middle-aged man who, when he was well, was mild-mannered and extremely intelligent and articulate. On this occasion he was raving. He stood in the middle of the ward brandishing a chair with which he was trying to hit me. He was enraged, incoherent, grotesque in his nakedness and madness. The other patients were horrified. They cowered behind the tables in the dining room where this miserable and humiliating scene was being enacted. This was not something that would be presented in a theatre or on film or in an opera. This was too grim and ugly; it was too awful.

More recently I attended a performance by a group of professional actors. Again the subject was madness. Again I had been consulted and assurances had been given regarding respect and authenticity, and again my tentative contributions were utterly and it appeared quite joyfully dismissed. The cast frolicked about in blissful abandon. The women shrieked and took off their clothes. The men masturbated with crazed determination. One character seemed to consider that this was all insufficiently mad and had stuffed a giant plastic phallus into his pants. Such was the energetic frenzy of his performance that the phallus became dislodged and the ridiculous object was flung onto the floor. This had a deflationary effect. The cast seemed momentarily to be embarrassed. The actor scrambled to reinsert the ludicrous encumberment back into his pants. The audience laughed. The performance thereafter seemed more muted, more stilted, as if the actors had become self-conscious and were unable to retrieve the liberating disinhibition of their caricatures of madness. It was dispiriting, but I suppose not disillusioning. It had happened so often before and I was not going to make any difference.

This disregard of the reality of mental illness, this disdain for the very phenomena that are ostensibly sought to be portrayed, is difficult to fathom. It is exasperating and hurtful to those profoundly affected by psychotic disorders in particular, and it is usually this group who are depicted in these lurid ways. Watching somebody have a panic attack is just not titillating or exciting or sufficiently dramatic. These representations also seem exploitative. The suffering of others is fodder for the amusement of the audience, and for the evocation of pity and fear and the consolation that one is not in such a way afflicted.

This circus of clichés and caricatures affords vicarious pleasures but also does harm. It is seldom that we read textbooks or scientific articles to inform ourselves about mental illness. Intentionally or not, we become informed by accounts in literature and film and theatre. We rarely bother to determine whether these representations are truthful. Of greater concern is the quality of the performances, or of the production, and whether we were moved or sufficiently entertained.

Agatha Christie's *The Mousetrap* is acclaimed as the longest-running play in the history of London's West End. It has probably reached hundreds of thousands. The dramatic tension arises from the mystery surrounding the identity of the murderer, who must be one of a small group of contenders. At the climax of the performance the murderer is identified by a policeman. This policeman, who appears to work as a psychiatrist on the side, declares the murderer to be 'obviously mad' before leading him away to be sedated and incarcerated. The perpetrator is quite obviously not mad, having planned the murders with great skill and forethought, and with understandable motivation. It is difficult not to think that many of the thousands who have attended this play will not have formed an impression that the criteria for madness must include the capacity for deceit and evil acts.

It is possibly naïve to think that the arts in general have any sort of responsibility, in particular a responsibility to educate. The arts are just a form of human activity. It may seem pompous to assume that there should be an obligation to fulfil any function at all. The arts reflect just one aspect of the exuberance of the marketplace, a response to the random flows of supply and demand, of fashion or the vagaries of intellectual discourse. One person seeks distraction, another to be informed, another excitement. We are all happily free to make our choices, and it is only in non-democratic or totalitarian systems where what we read and see and hear are determined for us, and this would be regarded as not art but indoctrination. This in itself is something of a caricature, but sometimes it can be helpful to consider a problem in terms of its opposing extremes, if only to find a feasible middle ground or compromise.

I am perplexed by the different experiences I have when attending a theatrical production, and what it might be that elicits these various responses. On one occasion I am bored, irritated, wishing I was somewhere else, and on another engrossed, stimulated, provoked into setting in motion my own train of thoughts. In one circumstance the proscenium arch seems rigid and alienating, in the other it disappears. In one production I am a spectator, in another a participant. In trying to understand my confused responses, it seems to me that being a mere spectator induces an unease, that being passive means being helpless or superfluous to whatever might be happening beyond the proscenium arch. In this situation I don't know what the point is of being there. There are no spaces to rethink or re-imagine or reflect. We are required to laugh or cry, or to be angry or awed. In these kinds of production we are also players, under direction, following a script, responding to cues, until or unless we become restless or disenchanted and disengage.

Another way is to cultivate the space. The book, the film, the play or the opera is a sort of proposal – a means, not an end in itself, of looking beyond or looking differently at the world so that circumstances do not seem to impose themselves upon us but provide opportunities to think and feel and behave differently, and possibly to be more free. The representations of madness in theatre can reinforce stereotypes and compound alienation and exclusion – or imaginatively and profoundly change accustomed and uncritical ways of thinking. I don't think it is naïve or idealistic to believe that the arts or humanities can also be of great value in changing perceptions about mental illness. With changed perceptions comes the hope of better understanding, and therefore improved care and inclusion.

With these possibly rather lofty and ambitious thoughts in mind I attended yet another performance of a well-known opera. It included what had come to seem an almost obligatory mad scene.

A grimly predictable portrayal was imposed on the audience. The lighting was dim and figures moved about in silhouette, seeking I suppose to create an atmosphere of a netherworld, a world of lost, abandoned souls. Figures in white gowns moved randomly about the stage like wraiths, animated at intervals by the familiar shrieks and jerks. It was I think intended to be horrifying or harrowing, but it was more like a pantomime. The persistence of these falsifying caricatures continues to confound me. It might be merely wishful to assume that there is any serious intention to portray mental illness in a realistic or respectful manner. Something else is going on; it seems possible that madness is being presented as a metaphor, or as a means of escape from a rational and a bleak reality.

In this respect, madness is imagined as liberating. Being mad you are free to express your deeper self, to give vent to your thrilling and dangerous passions. This conventionally seems to involve sex and violence. It is trite and superficial but also demeaning. If an artistic performance seeks to be taken seriously, if we take the trouble to go to the theatre in the expectation that we might learn something or be provoked into thinking about something in different ways, these thoughtless distortions are likely to lead to cynicism and a disenchantment with any notion of the potential value and importance of the arts. Theatre serves merely to distract and entertain. It is frivolous. It can make no useful contribution to the real world. Medicine and the arts are two different worlds.

The morning after this dismal experience, I set out to write what turned out to be a short opera or cantata with the title *Madness: Songs of Hope and Despair*. Anger and exasperation do not seem to be particularly worthy motivating factors; perhaps my attendance at that theatrical event was more of a precipitant of something I had wanted to do for some time. Certainly a central motivation was to create something that was authentic and respectful. At that stage I had no clear idea what that something was or what form it should take, other than that it should stand in emphatic contrast to the false and exploitative representations I had previously encountered.

Another related motivation arose from a frustration concerning the nature of the scientific perspective. Central to this are the necessary and valuable principles of objectivity, experimentation, verification and replication. These scientific methods have been of enormous benefit and provide the sound basis of modern medicine. A scientific foundation separates medicine from mere quackery. An objective stance is fundamental, but it seemed increasingly to me that it was not enough, and that valuable information was being lost or neglected by not including the subjective perspective.

Persons experiencing psychotic symptoms are not mere objects but subjects. Describing the terror of one's thoughts being stolen by a machine might validly be described as a persecutory delusion, but that seems insufficient. Merely ticking the boxes of a checklist of psychotic symptoms is an impoverished way of comprehending the rich and informative complexity of psychotic worlds. This objectivising stance neglects the experience of psychosis. It pays no heed to the meanings a person might attach to their symptoms, and to personal strategies of recovery. It seems excessively reductive to assume that because something is not quantifiable it is not real or meaningful.

A central idea was therefore that the voices of the patients themselves should be used. Confidentiality could be assured without too much difficulty by changing names and avoiding specific accounts that could identify individuals. I asked the permission of my patients. Without exception, they agreed enthusiastically. They did not seem overly concerned about the confidentiality issues. They said they wanted their stories to be told.

I had made previous attempts to describe first-person narratives but certainly in the mainstream journals little priority is accorded to qualitative studies, and my verbatim accounts seemed to me bland and prosaic. Literal records of patients' psychotic experiences somehow did little justice to the strangeness – and, at times, the surprising beauty – of their vivid, intensely lived, mad worlds. It seemed more possible that this might be articulated by moving beyond the conventions of theatre and integrating words with music and images, and so a collaborative project emerged.

In addition to the patients' voices it was important to include the other voices that contribute to the process of assessment and management in the acute phases of a psychotic illness, including the nurses, the doctor, the family, the lover. A neuroscientist, a traditional healer and a priest also sing songs that reflect the various and at times conflicting perspectives that form part of this turbulent process. A chorus is made up of patients and the nurses seeking to comfort them. The libretto tries to communicate the patients' confusion and fear and ambivalence, and also some of the anxieties and uncertainties of those seeking to help them. Both the music and the projected images aim to express the shifts in coherence and clarity and relative calm to chaos and disharmony and discordance. The natural inclination to find patterns or construct a meaningful narrative are deliberately disorganised. We sought to dislocate the senses and then establish fleeting moments of coherence to imagine madness.

There is no nakedness in the performance, no masturbation, no screaming and manic prancing about the stage, only a determined, respectful austerity. The intention is to describe in as authentic a way as possible the wide variation in the expression of psychosis, but also to evoke the sense of a mind in turmoil, to attempt to create a sense of what it must be like to be inside, to be there.

Madness: Songs of Hope and Despair was first performed at the World Psychiatric Conference in Cape Town in December 2016. There was acclaim. It was gratifying. Melodrama is superfluous and unnecessary.

I don't know if it will make any difference, but we tried.

23

Art and madness

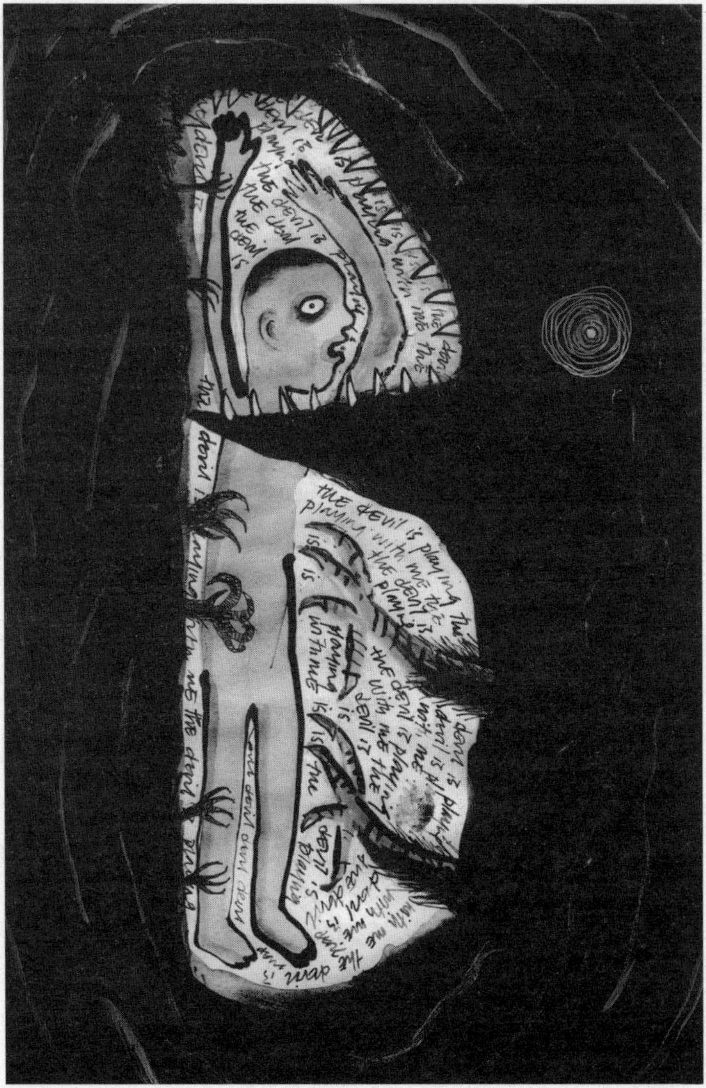

I have known Jonathan for years. He has a long, turbulent history associated with the hospital. In the outpatient clinic he tells me with some pride that he has been admitted on over thirty occasions. It has been some sort of battle, he says. He has been determined to demonstrate, most importantly to himself, that he is stronger than the illness. He would come in, get better, be discharged and then – to the dismay of all around him, including family and friends and ourselves – he would stop the medication and relapse and need to be readmitted yet again.

Now, he says, he is getting older. He is tired of this. He has lost too much. He is divorced and alienated from his children. He is unemployed and in poor health. He feels he has also lost his self-esteem and his confidence that he will beat this illness and regain control of his life. He is not depressed but he seems wearily despondent. He has now chosen to continue with the treatment. He tells me that he has not been readmitted for the past year – his longest period of remission since his first admission in his early twenties.

I feel a cautious elation. It is not too late. Despite many losses there is still a future. I suppose there is a reflex need for optimism, that the situation should never be considered to be beyond hope, and in Jonathan's remission there is a genuine sense of achievement and even in his middle age the possibility of a new beginning.

Jonathan was once a talented artist. When he is well he makes delicate, exquisitely crafted ink drawings, some of which he has given me and which I have proudly put up on the walls of my office. When he is unwell the nature of his art changes. He becomes more prolific, but the precision and clarity are lost. Lines become scrambled and entangled, the colours lurid, and over the images he compulsively scribbles reams of indecipherable prose and poetry. There is no sign at all of the graphic skill and the almost cold formality of the works he produces when he is well. He creates these mad works in an apparent frenzy and foists them on me with enthusiasm. On one admission he decides to transform his bed in the dormitory of the admission unit into an installation. He collects branches and bits of wire and string and other random objects that he finds in the grounds of the hospital and constructs an elaborate canopy over the bed. It is a ramshackle mess and requires considerable agility on his part simply to get access to the bed. I am deeply impressed that the nursing staff and cleaners allow this. The other patients are bemused, but despite their disorganised behaviour they make no attempt to interfere with this delicate and bizarre construction. There seems to be some shared acknowledgement that this is a project, a work in progress – and that, however incoherent, it is important for Jonathan.

His different, distinct ways of expressing himself seem to reflect in an eloquent way his shifting states of mind. It is not simply that when he is well his art is good and when he is sick his art is bad – not art at all, just incoherent ravings and scribblings. This elaborate, intricate, chaotic installation that he has constructed with such painstaking care in the ward suggests a quite desperate determination to give a three-dimensional form to something that is menacing and that could otherwise overwhelm him. He seems compelled. The task is urgent.

The finely executed drawings he creates when he is well seem to serve another function, to be necessary in a different way. There are in these images another kind of need, a careful imposition of order, of precision, of the clear demarcation of spaces. It is as if there are two different strategies for dealing with his madness. When he is ill in hospital, the spontaneous uninhibited process of giving form to inner turmoil with the hope of gaining control is in tension with the formal mastery he displays when he is well – a determination, having regained control, to maintain it, to keep at bay the disorder of psychosis.

Sitting together in the outpatient clinic we reflect on these past events and turn with some hesitation to the future. Despite his air of inertia and lassitude I feel the need to be if not naïvely optimistic, then at least positive. Circumstances have changed. There is no reason now to think that the past should repeat itself. At last there is a degree of stability. I urge Jonathan to take pride in what he has achieved in coming to terms albeit belatedly with his illness, and having now created the possibility of being free of the hospital and the dismal and surely soul-destroying routine of repeated relapses and readmissions. He is composed and thoughtful but there is an apprehension beneath the surface. In a way his struggle with his madness over many years is how he has come to see himself; it is part of his identity and now he wonders how he might adjust to this new world of relative order and calm.

We talk about purpose and direction, about finding new meanings and different ways of getting through the day and the rest of his life. Making art has also been part of his identity. Now there is an opportunity to work on his art without the disruption of his admissions to hospital. He could make use of his past experiences. He could creatively transform the misfortune and misery of so much that has happened to him into something possibly eloquent and helpful to himself and others. Making art is making a mark, a way of defining oneself and simultaneously reaching beyond oneself, marking the paper or the canvas and going through the surface to something beyond that is open and free. I imagine in this way that making art is an act of generosity and of hope, and for Jonathan, burdened as he is by the past, possibly some sort of liberation.

Jonathan looks at me as if from far away. He is quiet and then he sighs and says no, he does not think he can do that. It is not a feasible option. He implies in a polite way that I just do not know what he is up against, how difficult it has been for him and how difficult it continues to be. The struggle is not over. I ask him why not. He has not lost his skills. He has much to communicate that could be of great help to me in forming some understanding of his plight, but also to others in a similar position. More importantly, through art he could possibly give some form to the chaos: he might transform something distressingly without structure or discernible significance into something of value.

He responds almost vehemently. It is clear to me that he regards returning to making art as not good for him, that in some way it would be dangerous. He explains this with some difficulty but says that in order to make art – and this has been a pleasure for him – he needs to lose himself. Engaging himself in the process takes him away from himself, and nothing else matters. There has been a cost, and now he considers that cost too great. Madness, he says, is losing oneself in a way. In the past there was an almost joyful abandonment of the struggle to be sane, and he was able to regard his psychotic episodes as adventurous journeys. Now he believes too much damage has been done in the process. What he wants now more than anything else is some degree of peace and stability. But he knows this is fragile, and will always be. Making art, losing himself, would bring him too close to the edge or take him over it – something that now fills him with dread.

There is a sadness in this. I should have been relieved by his new determination to stay well, but in this caution there was a compromise. In choosing to become himself, not to lose himself in his madness, he has to put aside a vital part of himself.

The schizophrenia that Jonathan has struggled with for much of his life may be conceptualised as a disorder of the self. Defining the self is problematic and subject to a wide range of variables, including social and cultural factors. Being conscious of oneself, a degree of unity and stability, and internal and external worlds being separate are nevertheless fairly consistent features. In psychotic states this edifice breaks down. The sense of self or the integrity of the self fragments; the external world irrupts into the internal, essentially private world. In this respect there is an anguish or a crisis that is existential. Who am I in the world? Is the mad self or the sane self the true self, or is there a true self? I think Jonathan has found himself in this distressing quandary and is becoming exhausted by it. His task is now just to get through the days. Not only is the sense of self precarious but so is external reality. There is no continuity, no stability;

at any time the outside world could break down the feeble barriers and invade his inner world again.

The predicament that preoccupies Jonathan is characteristic of schizophrenia, but in other respects it is unusual. Some of the most disabling aspects of the schizophrenia spectrum are the neurocognitive deficits. These include impairments in the ability to imagine. To imagine is to be able to consider other possibilities, to be free of an obdurate, given state of affairs. It might be considered a basic requirement for being able to act on the world – to be an agent, not a passenger. This fails in persistent psychotic states. Many of our patients – to the greater distress of their families perhaps than of themselves – drift through their lives. I have tried repeatedly to persuade them if not to make art, at least to record what they have been through after emerging from a breakdown. I have had little or no success, and that is why Jonathan is unusual. I do not think this is because my patients are unwilling to oblige me, or that they might be afraid. I think it is because they cannot.

Madness: Songs of Hope and Despair was conceptualised as an attempt to give a voice to those suffering from severe mental illnesses. The question arises why a psychiatrist should presume to do this, and not the patients themselves and their families and communities. For the reasons I have attempted to articulate this was not possible. Perhaps the difficulty can be described broadly as an inability to find the necessary symbolic space. Using the utterances of my patients themselves and describing their stories was at least one way of being authentic and showing the necessary respect. For the same reasons we would have liked to use the art works of our patients for the project. Some were included, but regrettably few. We were attempting to get into the psychotic experience, to imagine it and communicate what it might be like. The very nature of the condition precluded us for the most part from using our patients' works.

In this there is a problem that I find perplexing. Dr Hans Prinzhorn, a German psychiatrist in the early part of the twentieth century, encouraged his patients to make art and collected their very various forms of art – including paintings, drawings and collages made elsewhere by patients in psychiatric hospitals throughout much of Europe. These extraordinary works have been widely published and presented across the world, and remain on permanent exhibition at the Psychiatric Clinic of the University of Heidelberg in Germany. The moving images eloquently convey the inner worlds of these patients. What has changed? Why, almost a hundred years later, has it been so difficult for us to find works of equivalent beauty and expressive power? There are I suppose many possible explanations: the art tutor might have encouraged a more conventional representational style in the belief that it might be therapeutic, and medication might have played some part. It is also possible that our patients today inhabit a different world, one with a plethora of images in a wide range of media, and that this might close down the spaces – even in the refracted worlds of the patients in our hospital – for making art that is furiously personal and profound and intensely meaningful.

I had previously tried to describe the subjective experiences of madness in more academically oriented articles, but the results seemed bland. For the cantata, integrating the libretto with music and with images – at times coherent and at others disorganised – brought the possibility of conveying more vividly and more forcefully the turbulence of psychotic states of mind. Fiona Moodie's art for the project created a sense of these shifting states of terror and stillness, of disorder and calm, eloquently and powerfully and more effectively than the work of any patient I have encountered. Hers is a work of art. It is reaching out, imagining, wondering. Otherwise there is nothing, only silence and empty spaces. I don't think that that is helpful.

I recently found myself wandering around a modern art gallery, trying to understand why I should be feeling so dispirited. Perhaps there was too much of it, perhaps I was in the wrong mood, but the works somehow seemed superfluous, attenuated, wilfully obscure and vapid. My impression was of a display of self-preoccupation, an almost solipsistic disregard for the confused world we inhabit in common. I felt like a mere spectator of a wan parade of introverted miseries. The works were accompanied by explanatory texts of dense jargon, replete with 'explorations', 'interrogations', 'discourses', 'narratives' and 'tropes'. Any notion of wonder – or sense of a need to communicate with clarity, or of caring deeply about a shared world – I suspect would have been regarded as sentimental and irrelevant. Perhaps I was also vaguely antagonised by the hallowed atmosphere of these large, antiseptic spaces, as if in denial of the banalities of fashion and the marketplace that drove the whole contrived process.

Perhaps I was also searching for the raw honesty and intensity and high risk of madness. The complex and confused – and at times contradictory – nature of Jonathan's artistic endeavours moved me profoundly, I think because they represented an urgent search and a yearning for meaning: a way of surviving and being in the world. I don't know which criteria are used to decide what might constitute good or significant art, but in some way what is valuable is the sense that it is necessary, authentic, disconcerting, and possibly dangerous.

24

Madness and machines

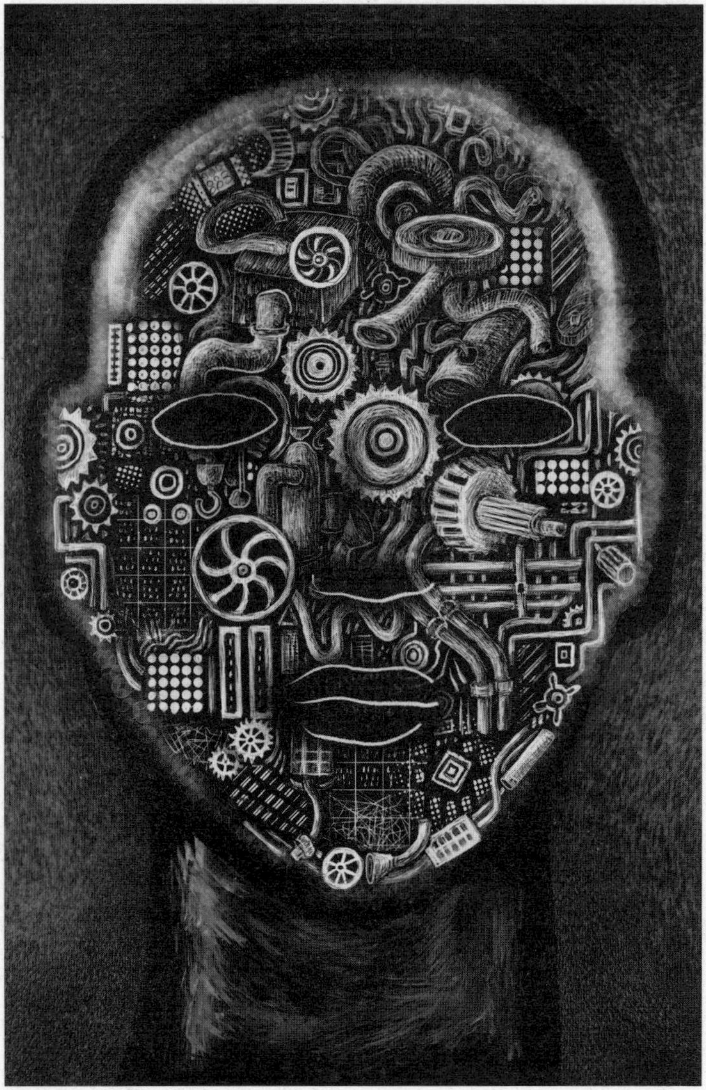

'It's my own brain that does it … it's like an electrical machine that switches on … when I'm well the machine has no control over me …when I'm ill the machine switches on … when you are well you've got control … you bring it on yourself … you think it's your subconscious and then this mechanism is triggered … if you are sitting in a chair and you want to get up before your time, you can't … it's hell.'

Ruben is describing the experiences that led him to an attempt to end his life.

We are in the outpatient clinic and he is explaining what happened. His brain was hijacked by a machine. Now he has recovered, and he speaks with great insight and eloquence about this terrifying experience.

I think he is speaking with insight because I have no idea what it must be like to feel that your brain is controlled by a machine. There is insight or an indication of recovery in that he associates the experience with being ill. The events are recalled with great clarity. There is no escape in forgetfulness. The experience is vivid. He seems to want me to understand. When he is ill there is no barrier, there is no distance, no capacity for abstraction that might enable him to interpret what is happening to him as a possible symptom of illness. He is so immersed in the experience that there is no space to question or doubt it. The nightmare is not simply that he has lost control, which may be something that many of us have experienced to some extent for short periods of time. In moments of high emotion and in states of grief or intense fear we might experience a fleeting sensation of having no control, or of the need and struggle to maintain control. What has happened to Ruben appears to be of a different quality. Not only has he lost control but that control has been usurped by a machine.

He could not attribute what was happening to him as something internal – an aberration that perhaps through force of will he might overcome. Any notion of personal agency had been cruelly and inexplicably surrendered to an external device, to remote control. There seems to be something particularly menacing about this experience of remoteness. This overwhelmingly powerful adversarial force was not close or tangible, yet it was intrusive and manipulative. It was mystifying to him. It had no shape. There seemed to be no substance to it.

Whatever it was, it was all the more sinister because he could not grasp it. He could not protect himself. He did not know what it was, so he could not devise strategies to defend himself. His psychosis had rendered him helpless.

It is imaginable, and again fleetingly, that we might feel that we are under the control of or unduly influenced by another – but this is 'as if', it is metaphorical. It does not equate to the concrete, anguished conviction Ruben describes. Being under the control of a machine is all the more menacing and degrading, an affront to human dignity.

This lack of any familiar element to which one might begin to attach meaning is described as a 'hell'. The malevolent machinery is relentless. It has switched off all meaningful signals, all familiar patterns and any hope of escape. It may be difficult to understand what might have been happening to Ruben in this psychotic and nightmarish state of being, but it is surely not too difficult to understand the desperation that led him to an attempt to end his life.

I had just taken up a post as a junior consultant when I first encountered David. I thought he might have been the superintendent of the hospital, or that he held some senior administrative position in the department. He had a dignified, urbane, detached demeanour. He was dressed immaculately. He was wearing a tweed jacket and a tie, his flannel trousers were ironed and his shoes were polished. He stood alone on the lawn, his hands clasped behind his back, gazing across the river and up towards the eastern buttress of the mountain. He seemed preoccupied but calm. Perhaps what was most striking about him was his stillness. I was often to see him in the same position, always alone, always absorbed in himself, always gazing outwards. It was unimaginable to me that he was a patient of the hospital. I did not know that he had been a patient for longer than any other, and that he was gravely ill. What was I expecting: torn, filthy clothes, swivelling eyes, wild hair, a raving lunatic?

The next time I saw David he was in the hospital clinic. At first I did not recognise him. He was emaciated. He was severely dehydrated. He appeared to be terrified. I thought he was close to death. The nurses were desperately trying to give him fluids and feed him but he was resisting them with a strange ferocity.

On that occasion he survived. He recovered and was eventually returned to his ward. I found him in his familiar position, restored to himself, composed, apparently intact.

It would never go away, he said. He was just waiting for it to start again and he did not know whether he would have the strength to cope with it. He was getting older and weaker. He was tired of it all. I had the impression that he was also tired of having to explain himself. Nobody really understood. Nobody could really help.

When he became ill, when he let down his guard, the machine would come on, he told me. At first it was insidious. He felt a vague disquiet, a sense of unreality, an uneasy and growing awareness that he was not quite in control of himself. This became more intense and eventually overwhelming. He could no longer resist it. He no longer had the strength. The machine had got to him, again. It was in total control. What surprised him, he said, was that he was surprised. When he was well it seemed impossible that this would happen again. It was inconceivable. Perhaps, he mused, this was just wishful thinking. Now he knew better. It would never go away, not completely. That was the last image I recall of David, standing alone, apparently impassive, gazing up at the mountain and towards the setting sun, waiting, I suppose, for it all to come raging back and engulf him.

However hesitantly it might have begun the control this machine exerted over him rapidly increased in its pervasive power. Initially it was just an almost dreamlike sense of disorientation, then a growing, sickening awareness that the machine was gaining control of his thoughts and actions. His helplessness filled him with dread. The machine bored relentlessly into his world, into the most intimate aspects of his life, and eventually into his body and his mind and soul. He became incapacitated. The machine controlled his ability to swallow, to feed himself, to breathe and to survive.

The horror of it, the absurdity and the monstrous injustice of it, was that this thing was being controlled by a homosexual couple living in London. He had never met these people. He did not know who they were or why they were inflicting this on him. He just knew with certainty that it was this couple who were controlling the machine that was controlling him. Perhaps it was just a random act of cruelty, perhaps it was to amuse themselves in some callous way. He could not explain it but what he knew with a fatalistic certainty was that it was real and that it had become unbearable.

David disappeared from the hospital a few weeks after this meeting. There had been no signs of a relapse. He had been his quiet, polite and reserved self. It seemed that, at least for the time being, he had regained some peace of mind. Now, abruptly, he was gone. There had been no indication that the machine was beginning yet again to exert its terrible control. He had never left the grounds before and we were all apprehensive.

The next morning I was informed by the hospital administration that the police had found his body washed ashore on one of the beaches on the other side of the city. There seemed to me something so utterly forlorn in the image of his crumpled, inert and always solitary figure, now dishevelled in death, beneath the glittering and impassive apartment blocks of the Atlantic seaboard. I do not know whether it had been due to the machine, and whether David had chosen not to tell us this time because it was hopeless, or whether it was his own decision finally to take control by choosing to end his life. I would like to think of this as an act of defiance, but it was probably and more simply driven by despair.

Machines – and more recently, specifically computers – loom large in the content of our patients' delusions. This is shaped to a great extent by cultural and probably socioeconomic factors. Believing that one's mind is being controlled by a computer is vastly more common in a middle-class, urban population, which very often corresponds with being white in our persistently racially preoccupied world. Our young black patients from rural backgrounds are far more likely to attribute their distress to witchcraft or the displeasure of the ancestors. It seems very probable – and there was some evidence of this emerging recently in our wards – that with urbanisation the wrath of the ancestors or the evils of witchcraft would be replaced by the cold and possibly more sinister malevolence of machines.

The prevailing theme has been the persecutory delusion of being under the control of a machine of some kind, but with recent and dramatic technological advances machines enter the world of psychosis in a very different way.

Machines are being created that are so intelligent that they are developing the capacity to learn or think independently. Mimicking human intelligence, these machines are beginning to surpass human intelligence. It is not unforeseeable and it is poignant that, at some point in the future, our much-vaunted consciousness will be a mere function of an algorithm devised by a machine that is without consciousness but is vastly more intelligent than ourselves, and that we won't know it.

Another implication of these advances is a possibility that in having minds of their own these machines will develop the capacity for madness.

It might provide a curiously informative perspective on our human madness to speculate on how a machine might go mad. A machine somehow seems unlikely to complain that it is being controlled by another machine. It is improbable that a machine would complain of being bewitched. Machines are unlikely to complain about hallucinations. They are unlikely to complain. They are more likely to go awry.

That might seem of little consequence. The machine no longer functions, or functions less efficiently. It is neither here nor there. It is simply a dud, a mad, useless machine. This fails to take into account the extent to which machines have crept into our humdrum lives. It might be an extreme position to claim that machines do control our lives – not in any metaphorical or insane way, but in the way of an increasingly and insidious dependence upon which we possibly choose not to reflect too much because of the clear and dramatic benefits. Technology has transformed our world, and one could only be a gloomy pessimist or a luddite or a doomsayer to dispute that this is not for the greater good. Yet those who have the knowledge and the expertise acknowledge that no program is entirely secure. A hacker with malicious intent can hack into any system and in this way powerfully disrupt food and water and power supplies, for example, and create havoc.

This does not necessarily require evil intent. It might merely require a fault, a glitch in an immensely complicated program, a machine gone haywire. It seems increasingly probable that a nuclear holocaust would be the outcome not of a battle between great powers, but of human error or an errant algorithm.

To some extent this scenario is analogous to the human brain and its malfunctions. Being the most complicated thing in the known universe the brain is in all likelihood more prone to error, however slight that might be. The problem arises that due to the very complexity of the system an error – however trivial – could have chaotic consequences. An apparently minor genetic variant, in isolation or perhaps acting in concert with some non-specific adversity in childhood or later exposure to cannabis, triggers a cascade of events that eventually manifest as schizophrenia.

A mathematical error in the engineering of a critical vault leads to the collapse of the cathedral. The higher the spire, the closer it reaches to heaven, the more precarious it becomes and the greater the risk that the whole edifice will come crashing down to earth. A broken string, a jarring note can change a symphony into a cacophony. A disconnection, or a disorganisation, of neurochemical transmission in a critical part of our brain may lead to the collapse of the infinitely complex and delicate construction of what we regard as ourselves and our sanity.

We are, it seems, ill at ease with this contingency, this embodiment of ourselves. It cannot be that our consciousness or what we believe to be the essence of who we are and what is intrinsic to our humanity could be so prone to chance and error. This might be a factor in the fear of madness, and the consequent stigma and the exclusion of those who suffer from mental illness.

We are afraid of our vulnerability. We are afraid of our being in part mere machines, things, bodies, and that fear is compounded by the knowledge that machines can, and often do, malfunction. This of course applies to any form of illness and is not confined to madness. It is understandable – surely not ridiculous and pathetic – and it is a reflection of a human fear of unavoidable death.

What is rather ridiculous and pathetic is that with advances in technology we come to believe that we will be able to achieve immortality. Whatever the means – whether we are frozen or the contents of our consciousness are uploaded into the blue skies of cyberspace – there is always going to be some bored and distracted technician who might momentarily fail to maintain sufficiently precisely the temperature or some software fault that brings the whole proud enterprise down to earth and to ashes. There appears to be no escaping our fragile dependency, and to think otherwise is illusory. The mind cannot escape the brain. We are bound to the machinery of ourselves.

Being bound does not entail being confined. While there might be a tension or some uncertainty as to who or what is in control, I do know that I do not feel as if I am a function of an algorithm, and that this is irreducible and uncontestable, whether or not at some other level of analysis it is illusory.

When our patients tell us they believe they are under the control of a machine, it seems possible that they are saying that in some way they are no longer under the illusion that they are in control. However frightening that might be, it is not madness.

Perhaps we are just machines anyway, with a degree of superfluous self-consciousness that we believe to be transcendent, granting us humanity. The question then arises whether in the process of evolution we are to become more or less like machines.

A teacher in my undergraduate years sought to explain the workings of the central nervous system by drawing a box with an arrow entering it at one end and another emerging from it at the other end. This represented the sensory input and the motor output. It became more complicated, with another box – or perhaps it was a circle – above the first box, representing higher control centres that regulated what the output should be if there were a multiplicity of inputs. This seemed ludicrously simplistic at the time but it has become intriguing in its ramifications. What if the capacity of this regulatory function became engulfed by an excess of inputs? Presumably the function would be referred upwards to a higher and more sophisticated regulatory centre. But what if at that level the system became overwhelmed again? Would the excess of signals, the surfeit of inputs or information, lose significance and become mere noise?

We live in a world increasingly preoccupied with information or data. We attach value to the accumulation of more and more information. We worship at the altar of big data. We believe that this will grant us greater control over the circumstances of our lives, or enable us to reach beyond ourselves. We need more and more information, and in the process there is the spectre of becoming bloated, rendered catatonic with an excess of information, gazing in a stupor at our screens, increasingly incapable of thought or action, drowning in helplessness. How to process the escalating torrent of information available to us in a useful way is not clear, but the predicament is a way of imagining madness.

25

Psychopathy and psychosis

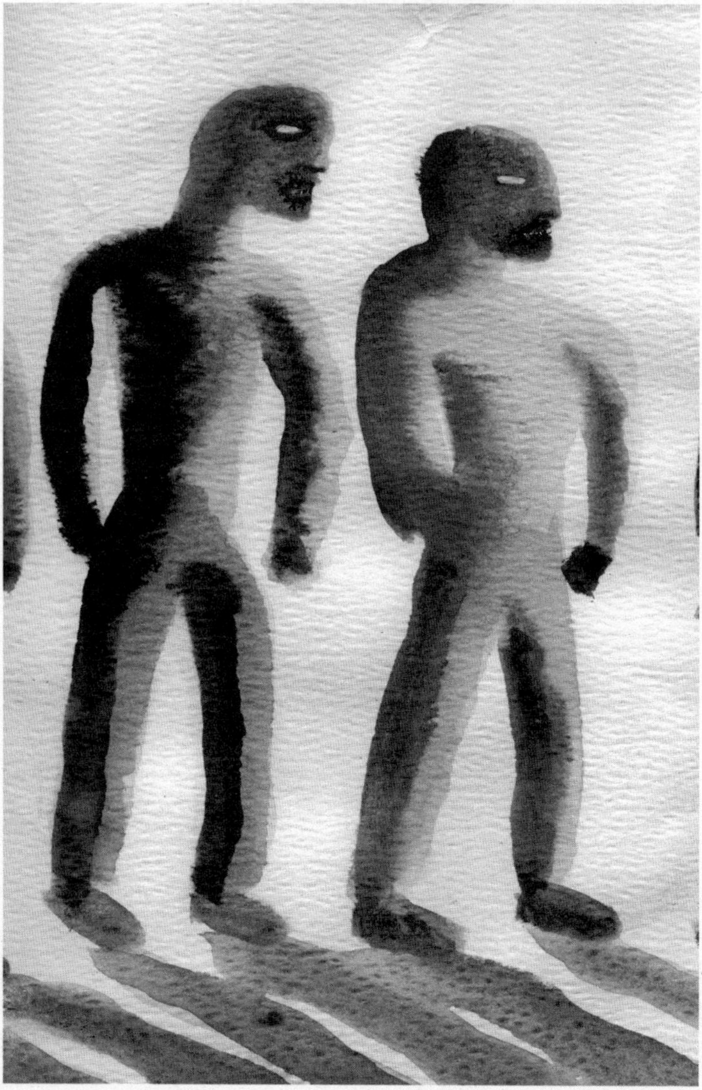

Psychopathy is not psychosis. The confusion of these two terms has contributed significantly to the burden of stigma. In the broadest possible terms psychosis refers to what might be described as a serious mental illness, or madness, and this includes the schizophrenia spectrum disorders, the more extreme expressions of the bipolar disorders and other neuropsychiatric illnesses, most commonly the dementias. Psychopathy is a particular form of personality disorder. As such it is enduring in its course rather than episodic and it is not associated with psychotic symptoms including thought disorders, delusions and hallucinations. Psychosis is regarded as an illness. Psychopathy is not. This itself is a source of much confusion and moral and legal debate and controversy.

A violent act is reported in the daily news. It is of such an extremely violent nature that notions of evil are invoked. The act was perpetrated in a 'psychotic frenzy', its cruelty and callousness are 'psychopathic'. Both terms in this context loosely and interchangeably define an extreme degree. The act is of such a heinous nature, it is so lacking in any human quality, that it can only have been perpetrated by a madman. Madness in this sense is not an illness. It is a form of behaviour beyond the human pale. It is incomprehensible. It is intolerable, it is unimaginable that a normal person could behave in this way. There has to be some explanation of this terrifying otherness, and all too often the explanation is madness.

This is 'psycho' territory, the domain of fiction, film and theatre, intended to thrill with horror. The extra syllables are of little consequence. Whether it is psychotic or psychopathic or even psychological is of lesser import than it being 'psycho', deranged, monstrous, bestial. The notion of something being psychological in this context itself evokes a certain unease. It is mysterious, uncontained and essentially private. It is beyond the reassurance of an objective or physical verifiability and therefore potentially dangerous.

In this morning's newspaper there is a report of a young man who has been declared a psychopath. The very nature of his crimes, the sheer gratuitous violence of his behaviour has led to this conclusion. It appears it is the action itself rather than the mental state that invokes the epithet or the diagnosis or the non-diagnosis. The judge asks whether this 'psychosis' is due to genetic or environmental factors. The young man's father is in prison following a conviction of murder. It is possibly careless misreporting, but the terms 'psychosis' and 'psychopathy' are used randomly in the report. It is assumed that it does not matter but it does. In the legal framework psychopathy is not an illness and the perpetrator is therefore considered criminally responsible for his or her actions. The consequence is in all likelihood a lengthy prison sentence, considering the extreme nature of the offence that has given rise to the notion of psychopathy. Psychosis is regarded as an illness. As such there is a high degree of possibility that whoever might have committed the act will not be considered criminally responsible, and will therefore be held in a hospital rather than a prison.

Mr Viljoen was a patient of mine many years ago. I remember him as a timid, sad and intelligent elderly man who had spent a large part of his adult life in the forensic unit of the hospital. He described the circumstances leading to his admission. It was so many years ago that he said his memory of the events preceding the tragedy was hazy. He was working as an accountant for a successful business in the city. He nevertheless recalled with clarity working one morning on a series of accounts with his manager. An entry was made by this unfortunate man of an account number that included a sequence of three sixes. The realisation then dawned upon Mr Viljoen that his employer was the devil. As a God-fearing Christian he concluded that it was his duty to rid the world of this evil person. He was not of a violent disposition and lacked physical strength, so he conspired with his nephew to kill the manager. This respected and prominent person in the community was thereupon hit on the head with a brick and died of the injury.

Both Mr Viljoen and his nephew were charged with murder. Mr Viljoen was indignant. Rather than being treated as a criminal he should be hailed as a hero, he said. He had destroyed the devil. He had saved the world. In the opinion of a forensic psychiatrist during the course of the trial he was considered to be delusional and as a consequence not criminally responsible for his actions. His nephew was not considered to be mentally ill. It is not known whether the notion of psychopathy was invoked at the time but he was considered to have acted cynically and with intent, probably motivated by the large amount of money that his uncle had promised him.

These events took place at a time when capital punishment was on the statute books. The young man was found guilty of murder and hanged. This caused outrage in the community. Two family members had conspired to commit the homicidal act. As a result one was cared for in a hospital and the other was dead. One was judged psychotic and the other treated as a psychopath, with the most dire consequences. This was considered a great injustice. That life-or-death decisions should hinge upon something as vague and abstract as a diagnosis of psychosis was regarded as a travesty.

Dmitri Tsafendas was found not to be criminally responsible for assassinating Hendrik Verwoerd. As some sort of compromise he spent most of the remainder of his life in prison and died eventually in a psychiatric hospital. This too caused outrage, particularly among the worshippers of Verwoerd. It was far too soft a way of dealing with a heinous crime. The tapeworm business was absurd, it was held – and anyway, regardless of whether the tapeworm or the man was ultimately responsible, Tsafendas should have been severely punished. Conversely, for those in vehement opposition to the policies of apartheid the attribution of the murder to madness robbed it of its political import.

Bartho was recently admitted to the unit after stabbing his friend in the neck with a kitchen knife. He also said that this was his duty. They were both in hell and this was a way of saving his friend. He told us that his last clear memory before everything became confused was the knife, which was under some form of external control, moving towards his friend's neck. He was dumbfounded. It was happening and it was not happening. He was a gentle person. Stabbing his friends was not in his nature. The knife in the neck of his friend, he said, was not 'poetic'. Now that he was getting better he believed his 'schizophrenic parts' were coming together, but he found being in the high care unit difficult because it was 'incoherent'.

Again it might not seem evident why this young man was admitted to a psychiatric hospital rather than being charged with attempted murder. A possible key is in his curious use of the word 'poetic', which suggested that this was a psychosis. It would be very unlikely that a psychopath would tell us that stabbing his friend in the neck lacked poetry, nor that he found the ward to be devoid of coherence. A more probable psychopathic position was that his friend was somehow asking for it and that he did not deserve to be in the ward among mad people.

The terms are not mutually exclusive. Psychopathy does not protect against psychosis. Younis has been admitted on numerous occasions, usually following acts of fairly extreme violence. This violence has in turn been precipitated by the use of tik, or methamphetamines. Younis knows the likely consequences of his methamphetamine use. He does not seem to care. He does not seem to have learnt anything from his previous admissions.

We convene a family meeting. An angry weariness hangs heavily over us. The mother is in tears. The family is devoutly Muslim. The son's delinquent behaviour has brought shame upon them. They have been ostracised by the community. The brother is hostile and impatient. On this most recent occasion, Younis had tried to throttle him. When asked why, Younis says he thought his brother was 'the king of calamity'. He says it was all because of the tik, which had made him 'crazy'. He shrugs and laughs. It's no big deal, he says. His brother has come to no harm and now that he has recovered it is time to go home. The mother weeps and says nothing. The brother says, 'He chooses to be like this. He knows what he is doing. He knows what will happen when he uses the tik. He enjoys it. He doesn't care. You are going to discharge him and it will be all right for a while and then he will start again and there will be violence. He is destroying our family.'

In the outpatient clinic I ask Younis why he continues this behaviour. Again he laughs. He is nonchalant. He blames his family. He says they no longer trust him. They cage him in, he complains. They treat him as if there is something wrong with him, or as if he is a child. They grant him no freedom. He gets bored. 'What is there to do, Doctor? Tik makes you strong. It is wild,' he tells me with relish. It all seems self-evident to him. He has come to live with the dire consequences, neither concerned nor deterred.

He is back in the unit a month later, roaring, berserk and exultant, his own king of calamity. 'Hey, Doctor! What did I tell you? It's mad, man. It's wild!' he shouts across the ward. He is chaotic and elated. He has stopped his medication yet again. It seems he does not understand the point of it, the grim struggle to be normal, the need to appease his family. He is bored and frustrated and angry. On this occasion he managed to obtain the keys to the family car and roamed up the coast not having any idea where he was going or what he wanted to do. The details are vague but he got involved in an altercation with a stranger. He assaulted this person; when the police were called he said he was our patient. He is not charged but brought back to the unit. When he greets me he shows no remorse. It has been a big adventure.

Younis did show many of the features of psychopathy in his lack of concern for others, especially his family, his failure to learn from his experiences and his careless disregard for the consequences of his actions. Yet I find myself surprised by a degree of sympathy for him. He is in an unenviable predicament. He is middle-aged and solitary and unemployable. He has alienated himself from his family and his community.

He is fully aware of the disgrace he has wrought upon them. He sees his life as empty, occupied only with the struggle to contain his bipolar illness and stay out of hospital. This saps his energy and demoralises him. It is not beyond understanding that he would rebel against these circumstances and take flight into mania, regardless of the predictable aftermath.

This conflict is not uncommon among people living with bipolar disorders in particular, and there is much debate about what is described as the comorbidity. The nature of the association of personality disorders with bipolar disorders is uncertain and the controversies are about whether the one group is integral to the other or whether the one predisposes or is a consequence of the other. The difficulties might arise in part from the nature of psychiatric diagnoses – and in particular the hazy construct of personality disorders. There is something inherently problematic in making a diagnosis of a personality disorder that is not considered to be a mental illness, and more specifically not an illness in a medico-legal sense, in that somebody with a diagnosis of a personality disorder is considered responsible for his or her actions. A further complication or uncertainty arising from this is what to do. A diagnosis implies a problem that requires a solution. The treatment of personality disorders is controversial, and this concerns – among many other issues – whether treatment is either beneficial or even warranted.

It is not clear how the diagnosis of a personality disorder is useful or helpful. The problems are compounded by the pejorative associations of the diagnosis or the construct. Particularly with regard to psychopathy or the antisocial personality disorders, the implication is that the behaviours that prompted this assessment are morally reprehensible and the character of the person diagnosed in this way is deeply flawed and beyond help. With regard to the newspaper report mentioned above, the recommendation to the court was that the perpetrator was dangerous, that he was unlikely to benefit from rehabilitation, and that he was likely to reoffend on release – and that therefore he should be given a lengthy prison sentence.

Not infrequently in our unit, when called upon to assess a patient on admission, and usually in the context of an act of violence, the registrar would conclude in the absence of any clear psychotic symptoms that the patient was 'just a psychopath'. This was dismissive. The message was that there was nothing for us to do. He, or more rarely she, belonged elsewhere – usually prison.

I rarely encountered a patient in our unit with a diagnosis of a personality disorder who had not been profoundly damaged by life circumstances. These extreme behaviours did not arise from nowhere. The usual trajectory was from a broken home, an absent or abusive father, a neglectful mother and a total absence of any form of support or nurturing, to a profound lack of self-esteem and a grim descent into drug abuse, gangsterism and criminality. These patients, and that is how they were described while in the unit, provoked an anger and a moral indignation that too often deflected attention away from the tragedy of these abject histories.

There are of course exceptions, but I struggle to recall any in my own clinical experience. A deeply moving and harrowing account is given in a memoir by the mother of one of the young men involved in the Columbine High School killings in the USA. She describes a loving, supportive, relatively privileged and – she uses the word carefully – normal family. There were no clear antecedents to an act of extreme brutality. The mother agonises over these events in painful detail. She is unable to explain her son's behaviour. The killings are terrifyingly unfathomable. This is another kind of psychopathy.

The difficulties in the diagnostic construct of personality disorders relate to the problem of the notion of personality itself. The way we are is probably more random and contingent than we would like to think. I do not know how I would be without the good fortune and the many chances that have been afforded me.

I doubt if I would be the person I am if I had been born into impoverished circumstances, been abused by my parents, left school early and had no prospect of a job, and lived without any self-respect and any hope.

26

Fear

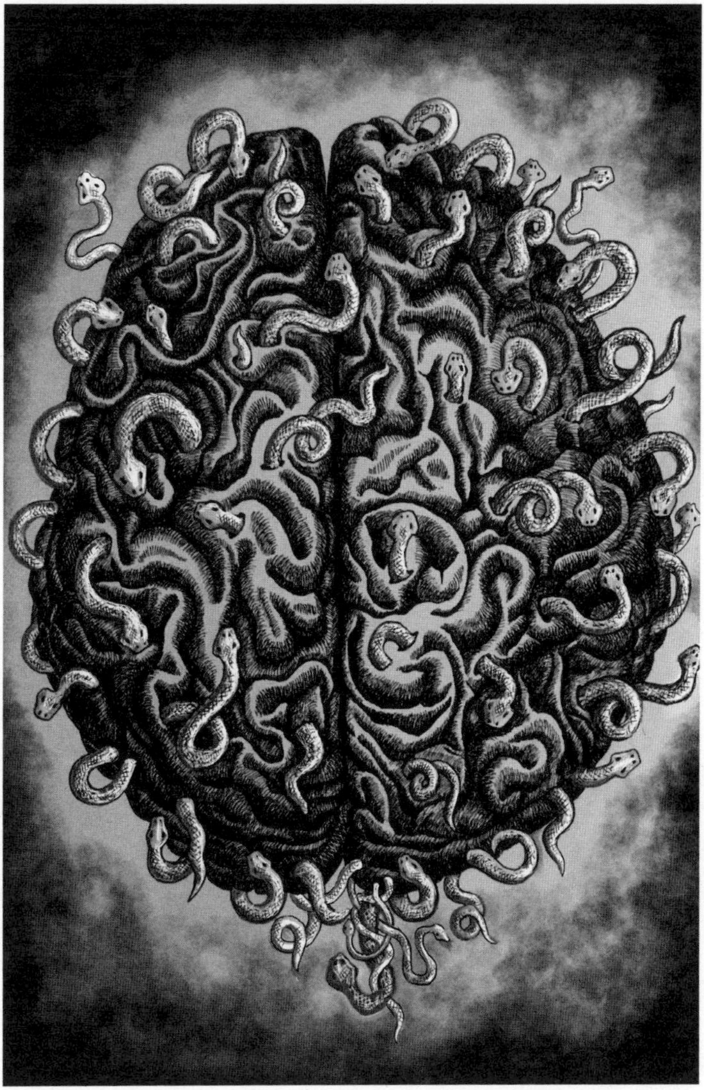

Fear pervades madness. Being mad we fear the world. Being in the world we believe to be sane and ordered we fear madness.

Wynand has disappeared. It is now three weeks since he left the boarding house where he has lived since his discharge from our unit about a year ago. His mother is in my office. She is in tears. 'Do something, Doctor. You have to find him.' There have been various sightings of him. He has been seen rummaging in refuse bins. He is described as gaunt, dishevelled, raving to himself. At every attempt to apprehend him, he has fled. 'Do something, Doctor! He needs help. He needs to be in hospital. I can't stand this. He is going to die. You have to do something.'

The manager of the boarding house reports that he probably stopped taking his medication about a month ago. The problem is compounded because he has tuberculosis and it is almost certain that he has also stopped that medication. It is winter and it is difficult to imagine that he will survive much longer if he is not found. He frightens people. It is more likely that they will close their doors than help him. Occasionally a call is made to the hospital to report that he has been seen. By the time the police arrive he has disappeared. The police are reluctant to accord this a priority. There are other, graver crises to which they have to respond. This is not a criminal matter, they tell me.

The mother is distraught and inconsolable. The people in the community are afraid. He is roaming the streets and he is unpredictable and they think he might be dangerous. I do not know his state of mind but it is difficult not to think that he is afraid. It is usually fear that drives this behaviour – a concrete fear of an imagined danger, or something more diffuse and inescapable, the threat of danger being everywhere, of there being no refuge.

I am afraid. I cannot console or reassure the mother. I am afraid that her fears might be justified and we might not find him and that he will die. He is vulnerable and unable to look after himself. He could die of exposure, his disorganised behaviour could provoke a homicidal assault, he could succumb to the tuberculosis. Anything is possible and nothing is certain.

Andries is wailing and howling and screaming in the ward, causing the other patients great distress. 'Oh my God, oh my God, oh my God!' he cries. He is inconsolable and it is a struggle to understand what might be the cause of his torment. One part of it seems to be that he believes he has to leave, and that by keeping him we are only making his predicament more intolerable. Eventually a nurse manages to coax him into a quiet corner and gain some understanding beyond the mostly incoherent moaning and shrieking. It still does not make much sense, but it becomes apparent that he believes his family has been killed, or that he has killed his family. He knows and accepts that the community will kill him in revenge. The only option is for him to kill himself, either to pre-empt the horror of his own impending murder or to punish himself for his dreadful crime. We are cruelly making everything worse for him by confining him to the ward. We don't understand. We are not helping him. On the contrary, we are hindering him from doing what he has to do. He has no choice. He is doomed.

It seemed to me that the worst kind of fear, the most intense and the most intolerable, was the fear that had no form or shape or meaning. These patients were utterly immersed in their fear. They could provide no explanation of it, they had no understanding of its source and they certainly had no idea what to do about it. Fear rendered them catatonic.

The nurses describe Zenzele crawling around the edges of the ward, groaning in terror. They ask him what the matter is but he just mutters incoherently and weeps and moans and sighs. He gnaws at his fingers and blood drips in bright streams from his mouth. The other patients are horrified. Everybody wants to help. 'What is it, Zenzele? What's going on? There is nothing here. There is no danger. Why are you so afraid? What are you seeing that we cannot see?' He casts his eyes about in panic and confusion. Eventually, almost to himself, unsure, he mutters, 'The snakes, the snakes are coming at me.' It seems he is desperate for something, anything, to account for the terror that is overwhelming him. The snakes might be quite random, but they provide some kind of an explanation. They are a start, at least. He knows about snakes. Snakes are out there in the world. He has seen snakes before and snakes are a recurring theme in his cultural, mythical world. You could also do something about a snake, like hitting it on the head. Slowly, faltering, Zenzele calms himself and regains his composure. Later, 'What snakes?' he says, bemused.

Anxiety, and also fear, we can for the most part understand. These states of mind can be considered appropriate and serve a function. A degree of anxiety for example can be useful in motivating us to prepare for an exam. If we cannot swim it is helpful and quite possibly life-saving to be afraid of water. The problem arises when states of fear and anxiety are not appropriate, or utterly disproportionate, or there is no context for making sense of these powerful and potentially chaotic feelings. Fear and anxiety can then feed upon themselves. The problem escalates and panic and terror ensue.

We have no idea what triggered the extreme response we observed in Zenzele. Some spark was ignited, some switch was pulled, there was some idea, there was some neurochemical turbulence that suddenly and wildly spun out of control and overwhelmed our young patient. I tried to imagine it, Zenzele, his fist crushed into his bleeding mouth, staring in paralysed horror at something vast and evil towering above him and swaying with menace, something undefined that could have been a snake or a writhing mass of snakes, maybe hissing, a tongue or maybe many flickering, vast fangs flashing, gleaming hateful eyes intent on his destruction. I could not imagine it. It is not possible to enter into another's mind, but we can make inferences from the behaviour we observe and I think we were all distressed by the mad and intense distress we witnessed that afternoon in the admission unit.

The neurobiology of fear is to some extent understood. A threat in some form is perceived, and in very broad terms two systems are activated: one rapid and more or less unconscious and mediated at lower levels of the central nervous system, the other slower and conscious and mediated at higher levels.

A decision whether to fight or take flight makes sense in terms of a very basic need to survive, but the various cognitive and emotional and other factors that shape that response are complex and cannot simply be assumed to be the most effective or efficient in that specific context. Fear becomes pathological when this system goes haywire. The very mechanisms intended to protect turn awry, and we become incapacitated. An innocuous event is misconstrued as menacing.

This in itself can be due to a host of factors, including past experience and a current disposition of mind. Being fearful, on guard, we become more fearful, more wary, more inclined to perceive danger. Lower brain centres are activated and the body goes into a state of high alert. Adrenaline flows through the system. Our hearts beat faster, our breathing is shallow and rapid, we might become dizzy and nauseous. Rather than informing an appropriate course of action, the more immediate, visceral, intensely powerful, emotional – possibly blunter – response can overwhelm the slower, more elaborately calibrated, evaluative system. We become paralysed with fear. We lose a sense of control and panic ensues. Our thoughts are distorted and we become disorganised by fear. In this frenzied state of mind we cannot respond to reason. We become inconsolable. Zenzele could not hear us. He was overwhelmed by terror.

Last night, taking the dogs outside into the garden I misjudged a step in the dark and I fell. I found myself lying on my back, gazing up at the stars, momentarily disoriented. I thought very briefly that I might have done myself harm but quickly reassured myself that I could move all my limbs. I was all right, I told myself, but my body did not seem to heed this. I began to shake violently. I found it difficult to breathe, my heart seemed to be beating dangerously fast, and a curious, deeply unpleasant electrical sensation suffused my whole body.

This must have lasted only a few seconds, but during that time I felt I was out of control; it was this rather than any fear of having done myself harm that scared me most. My body seemed to have developed a mind of its own. My attempts to reason with myself that there was no danger, that it was just a careless accident and that there was no cause for alarm, seemed for that short while feeble and inadequate. My sense of myself had become disorganised: one self was telling me that that I was all right and in control, and another – more embodied – self was sending me very clear signals that I was most emphatically not all right. I was in the grip of a violent, wholly disproportionate physical response over which my conscious, rational self seemed for those frightening moments to have no control.

Anxiety and fear are necessarily and inevitably part of our lives. The problem then might arise less from the nature of the stimulus itself and the perceived danger than from the inappropriateness or the disproportion of the response and the wrongful or misconstrued interpretation of the context. Zenzele appeared to be in great fear, and it seemed possible that he formed the idea of the snake or of those many snakes to account for this fear – or at least to start the process of mitigating the fear by giving it some form. I soon forgot about my wildly disproportionate response to a minor fall. It seemed ridiculous. It was unimaginable that Zenzele would ever be able to consider his fears ridiculous.

We could not reason with Zenzele while he was in the throes of terror. In this circumstance, the quickest and most practical way of alleviating his distress was to use medication. A simple benzodiazepine is an effective way of diminishing the incapacitating distress, enabling one to regain a degree of control and restore at least some sense of proportion. Only then might it become possible to use reason to dismantle the looming towers of fear and terror, to put things hopefully into some sort of perspective and to restore at least a semblance of calm.

A young medical student made a particular impression on me during the various ward rounds and seminars that students are required to attend. She was inquisitive and bright and thoughtful, and at some stage I found the time to ask her whether, given her clear interest in the subject, she would consider specialising in psychiatry once she had completed her undergraduate studies. She said she had given this some thought but had decided that it would not be suitable for her. She did not think she would be able to cope. I was surprised, and asked why she should think in that way as she appeared to be a remarkably mature and confident young woman. She said she was fearful. But is that not just part of being a medical student, or a doctor? I argued. You cannot not be anxious if you have any imagination.

It is a source of amusement to senior doctors to observe students in whatever speciality they might be engaged believing that a chest pain signals imminent cardiac arrest, a mere cough treatment-resistant tuberculosis. When we qualify and become doctors a fear that we will miss a diagnosis, that we will make a surgical error or that we will not be able to help seems an inevitability.

'No,' she said, 'it's not that.' She seemed to struggle to articulate what she wished to say. 'Perhaps it's got something to do with my young age, but it's too close. I find myself at times identifying with the young patients on the ward. I become frightened that this might happen to me. I find myself avoiding these encounters and that is not helpful. I don't think I could be a psychiatrist.'

I am also fearful at times, but not to the extent that I have considered turning back as I cross the river to enter the hospital and rather flee to the mountain. It is less the fear of not being able to help, I think, than the fear of becoming insane. The loss of the feeling of being in some control, however precarious that might be, and of the sense of the world as having some meaning or stability has filled me on many occasions with dread. Turning away from this – turning back – neither helps nor dispels the fear, and perpetuates the exclusion that seems to be so much a part of the suffering of madness.

We can all help. One way might be if not to overcome our fears, at least to resist the temptation to turn away, and to be there and listen and in this way contain the fear by giving it some form and meaning, restoring a degree of proportion and hopefully bringing some calm.

27

Anxiety, psychiatry in disarray and a celebrity circus

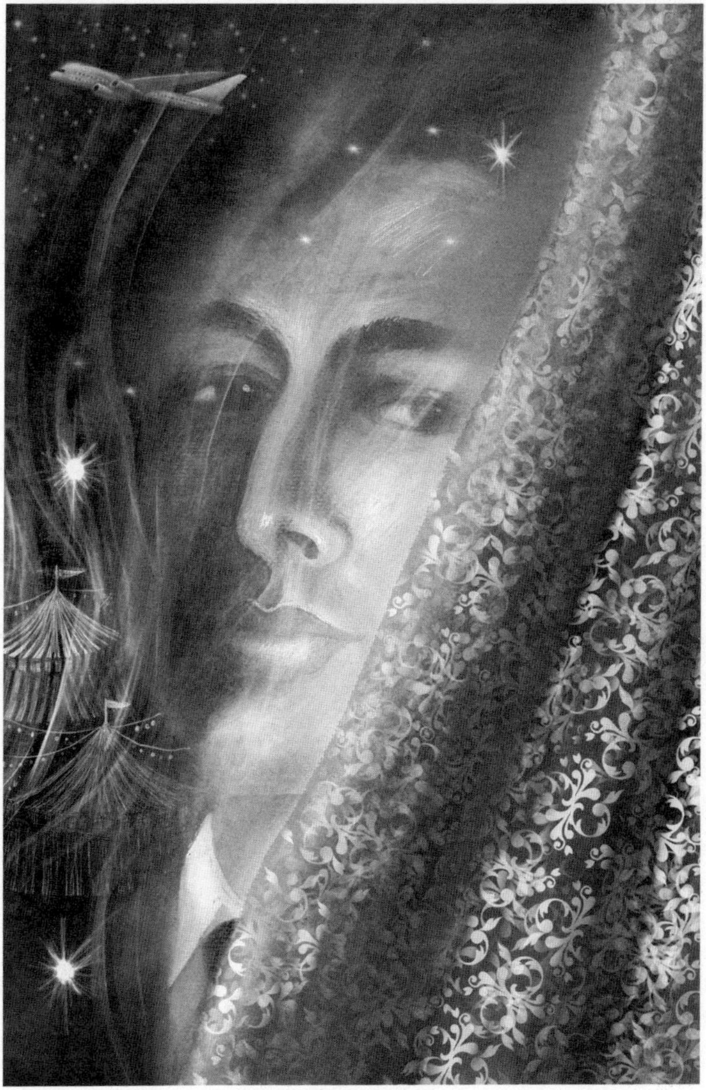

It is 7 November 2010. A beautiful and glamorous couple arrive in Cape Town on their honeymoon. He is a wealthy businessman from Bristol in the UK and she is an engineer of Indian origin, resident in Sweden. Last month, they celebrated their marriage at a three-day Hindu wedding attended by five hundred guests in Mumbai in India. They leave shortly thereafter for South Africa. They take a domestic flight to the Kruger National Park where they stay in a luxury lodge for four days, returning to Cape Town International Airport on 12 November. There they engage the services of a taxi driver to take them to the five-star Cape Grace Hotel. They retain this driver as a tour guide. The next evening he drives them through the city to Strand on the False Bay coast where they have a light meal.

On the way back to the hotel, the wife is reported by the husband to say that she wants to see 'the real South Africa'. The driver takes them into Gugulethu, a township on the outskirts of the city notorious for its high crime rate. Shortly after the driver turns off the main road, two armed men hijack the taxi. After driving a short distance the driver is thrown from the vehicle. The husband is robbed of his wallet, his watch and a mobile phone. After driving onward for about twenty minutes he is also thrown from the car. On the morning of 14 November in Lingelethu West the young wife is found dead on the back seat of the abandoned taxi. She has suffered a single gunshot wound to the neck. The body is removed to a city mortuary where this gunshot wound, having severed an artery, is confirmed as the cause of her death. There is no sign of a sexual assault. On 17 November her body is released by the South African authorities and she is returned to the UK, accompanied by her husband.

The murder makes global headlines. In the UK, the *Daily Mail*'s website runs the story under the headline 'Honeymoon horror: Newlywed Briton's wife killed after robbers hijack them in taxi'. The high rate of crime in South Africa again receives international attention. On 20 November the taxi driver is arrested. Reports begin to emerge that the killing had been planned, that it was not just another random hijacking that had gone terribly wrong. The driver reports that he had been paid R15 000 for the murder. On 7 December the husband, Shrien Dewani, is arrested in Bristol under a South African warrant on suspicion of conspiring to murder his wife Anni. On 8 December, Dewani appears in a City of Westminster Magistrates' Court. He is remanded in custody as South Africa prepares for his extradition. It proves to be a long and fraught process.

In arrests made soon after the murder, hijackers Mziwamadoda Qwabe and Xolile Mngeni and hotel receptionist Monde Mbolombo admit to their involvement in what they initially claim was an unintentionally fatal robbery and kidnapping. Confronting the likelihood of life in prison, they later change their account of events to allege that the crime had been a premeditated murder at the behest of Anni's husband Shrien Dewani. The taxi driver, Zola Tongo, initially claims to have been an innocent victim. Faced with the evidence against him in which the co-conspirators implicate him, he also changes his account and alleges that the husband was the instigator of his wife's murder. All those implicated at this point in the killing of Anni Dewani have lied to the court. It is hardly credible that the case against her husband should be based on the testimonies of these clearly unreliable key witnesses.

In December 2010 British police question a German male escort or prostitute, Leopold Leisser. He calls himself the German Master. He claims to have been in regular contact with Shrien Dewani for months before the crime. He tells the authorities that their encounters involve sadomasochistic sex. Dewani reportedly has to lick his boots. The German Master is to be the next key witness in the case for the prosecution.

Plea bargains are offered to the accused in exchange for future testimony in legal proceedings. Zola Tongo pleads guilty to murder in December 2010 and is sentenced to eighteen years in prison. Mziwamadoda Qwabe pleads guilty to murder and is sentenced to twenty-five years. Xolile Mngeni is convicted on a charge of murder and is sentenced to life in prison. Monde Mbolombo admits his involvement in the crime, but is offered immunity in exchange for testimony against the others alleged to have been involved in the crime. In July 2014 a medical parole application is made on behalf of Mngeni, who is reported to be terminally ill owing to a brain tumour. Parole is denied and he dies in prison in October 2014. The German Master is found hanged in his Birmingham apartment in November 2016. His suicide is attributed to stress relating to the adverse publicity arising from his involvement in the case against Shrien Dewani.

On 8 February 2011 Dewani's legal team file papers setting out the grounds on which extradition to South Africa is to be opposed. He is said to be too ill to be extradited. The nature of his illness is vaguely described as a 'stress-related condition'. That month, he is admitted to the Bristol Royal Infirmary. A provisional diagnosis is made of a post-traumatic stress disorder (PTSD). There is an unconfirmed report of an attempted suicide. Anxiety and depression emerge as key factors in this sequence of events. His condition appears to deteriorate and in April he is compulsorily detained under the Mental Health Act 1983 at Fromeside Clinic in Bristol.

In May the extradition hearing begins at the Belmarsh Magistrates' Court in London. Dewani's barrister, Clare Montgomery QC, argues that the extradition proceedings are hanging over her client 'like the sword of Damocles' and that he needs a period of calm to recover from the symptoms of anxiety and depression and to prepare himself for extradition. She argues that a twelve-month period under medical treatment would increase the speed of her client's recovery, rather than jeopardise it – as it would be if he were to be sent to South Africa. He is reported to be making a slow recovery. One damaging factor is said to be his 'constant awareness of the court proceedings'. The court is informed by his psychiatrist that the symptoms are of a moderate to severe degree and that he continues to pose a suicide risk. The court also hears that Dewani 'is unable to give an account of himself, possibly because he cannot remember', which is a curious supposition given that intrusive memories are a central feature of PTSD. The section order in terms of the Mental Health Act 1983 is renewed.

The state of Dewani's mental health becomes increasingly central to the repeated postponements of his extradition to South Africa. Initially the symptoms are described as an 'acute stress disorder' and a 'depressive adjustment disorder'. This is revised to a PTSD and a 'clinical' depressive disorder. His counsel describes difficulties in communication with her client and tells the court that his continuing ill health prevents her from taking instructions from him. These are not characteristic features of either anxiety or depression.

It is further submitted on behalf of Dewani that 'if it is true – and it plainly is the case – that Mr Dewani is seriously mentally ill, and he were sent back to a prison system that simply cannot cope with that level of mental illness, that is a violation of articles 3 and 4 of the European Convention of Human Rights which prohibits inhuman or degrading treatment'. The trial of Shrien Dewani for murder becomes a trial of the South African prison services. It also becomes a challenge to South African medical services.

In a report by two eminent British psychiatrists submitted on behalf of Dewani it is stated:

> This risk would be unacceptable in the absence of proper and adequate management of his illnesses. The prognosis for recovery depends on whether Mr Dewani can receive treatment. If he cannot then the prognosis is poor … travel to South Africa would greatly enhance his distress and cause him substantial further psychological harm. It may result in him killing himself … the problem with extraditing him now is that even with the best possible psychiatric facilities in South Africa it will be very difficult to get him to a state where he is fit to plead.

The report concludes that 'there is no doubt that Mr Dewani suffers from a severe and incapacitating mental illness. He is not faking the symptoms. There is currently a real and significant risk of suicide. That risk will increase if he is extradited to South Africa'.

The High Court in England temporarily halts Dewani's extradition on the grounds of poor mental health. The court rules that it would be 'unjust and inappropriate' to send him to South Africa immediately, but rejects claims that he should not be extradited on the grounds of human rights. It declares that in the interests of justice he should be extradited 'as soon as he is fit'. Ashok Hindocha, the uncle of Anni Dewani, says after the hearing that the family desperately needs answers. He says, 'I don't know how much longer the family members can take the pressure psychologically.'

In addition to concerns raised about Dewani's mental health, doubts are expressed on behalf of Dewani regarding the likelihood of a fair trial in South Africa. The South African police chief, General Bheki Cele, says, 'A monkey came all the way from London to have his wife murdered here … he thought we South Africans were stupid when he came all the way to kill his wife in our country. He lied to himself.'

In March 2014 the High Court in England finally rejects all grounds to appeal against extradition and denies Dewani the chance to take the case to the appeal court. The court accepts the validity of an undertaking on behalf of the government of South Africa that if Dewani is not fit to stand trial within eighteen months he should be returned to the UK. With regard to the forthcoming case in South Africa, the Hindocha family say, 'We need it … South Africa needs it … the world needs it … everybody wants to know what happened to Anni … everybody is seeking justice for her.'

Shrien Dewani is extradited to South Africa on 7 April. He arrives at Cape Town International Airport on 8 April on a chartered flight, accompanied by a doctor and nurse and a bevy of officials. He is arrested and immediately taken to court where he is charged with five offences: conspiracy to commit kidnapping, robbery with aggravating circumstances, kidnapping, the murder of his wife and obstructing the administration of justice. He pleads not guilty to all charges and is remanded to Valkenberg Hospital for the assessment and treatment of his psychiatric problems. He arrives in a cavalcade of vehicles with the international press in attendance. It is a circus. Shrien Dewani, grotesquely, is a celebrity. He is also now my patient.

Given this history and the global attention being paid to the saga, it was of critical importance but also difficult to keep a determinedly open mind and to be impartial and rigorous in our assessment. I could not ignore but I could not allow myself to be swayed by the opinions of our respected and esteemed colleagues in the United Kingdom. Our multidisciplinary team interviewed him and observed him and, over the weeks and months he was with us, evaluated him with I think the greatest care possible. I began to form an opinion but made a strenuous effort to not allow my thinking to influence my colleagues. Nevertheless, a consensus did begin to emerge.

I cannot describe in any detail my encounters with Mr Dewani in regard of the professional code respecting confidentiality in the doctor–patient relationship. I can, however, summarise a report I submitted to the court as this is in the public domain. With the support of the multidisciplinary team, I developed the opinion that Mr Dewani was not suffering from any form of mental illness and that he should therefore be discharged from our unit. I am not sure what Dewani might have been thinking, but I was not prepared to allow him to stay in our system for eighteen months only to return to the UK being considered unfit to plead owing to mental ill health.

In the report, I wrote:

> At the time of admission Mr Dewani presented as being calm, alert and cooperative. His manner was confident and self-assured. He

showed no features of anxiety and depression. He denied suicidal thoughts … he insisted that his intention was to appear in court to face the charges against him and that he wanted no further delay in the proceedings. Owing to the low risk he presented he was transferred to a medium-security unit. During the following weeks his confident demeanour diminished. He appeared more anxious, particularly during more formal interviews, and at times showed hypervigilant behaviour, flinching dramatically in response to the routine noises of a busy ward. He was distracted by these external stimuli but was able to rapidly regain the focus of attention. The occasional symptoms of anxiety, tearfulness and depression were considered understandable in the context of his failed appeal against extradition and the pending court appearance. At other times, in interactions with the occupational therapist and the clinical psychologist, or when unaware of being observed by the nursing staff, he appeared more calm …

> … The medication prescribed in the UK was gradually withdrawn owing to the unclear benefit and side-effects including irritability and anxiety, impaired concentration and biochemical abnormalities. At the time of writing Mr Dewani is on no regular medication. The anxiolytic prescribed on an as-required basis at the time of his admission has not been used …

I reported that a consensus had developed among the members of the multidisciplinary team that Mr Dewani was not depressed. With regard to the diagnosis of PTSD I stated that, while it was acknowledged that Mr Dewani did appear to meet the standard criteria for this diagnosis, the context should be taken into account in that the symptoms of anxiety could more probably be accounted for by his predicament at the time rather than past events. The avoidance displayed could be less an inability to recall past traumatic events than an understandable anxiety with regard to needing to appear in court to account for the circumstances leading him to be charged with the murder of his wife. For these reasons, the diagnosis of PTSD was set aside. I reported: 'At the time of writing the opinion is that Mr Dewani is not suffering from a mental illness. It is recommended that Mr Dewani should be discharged from this unit. Further hospitalization is unlikely to benefit him and on the contrary is more likely to have the adverse effect of reinforcing the avoidant behaviour that has developed subsequent to the events of November 2010.'

On 6 October 2014, after a delay of over three years following the charges of murder against him, the trial finally commences in the Western Cape High Court. Under cross-examination the key witnesses who alleged Dewani's involvement contradict their previous statements and one another on most of the central elements of the 'murder for hire' story. The testimony of the German Master is judged to be irrelevant. Dewani's sexuality was not considered to be on trial. On 24 November, after the closure of the case for the prosecution, Dewani's counsel argues for the case to be dismissed citing a lack of credible evidence linking her client to the crime. On 8 December this application is granted. Dewani is acquitted of all charges against him. He boards a flight for the UK.

The presiding Judge Traverso says in court that the evidence of the three criminals already convicted of murder was 'so improbable, with so many mistakes, lies and inconsistencies you cannot see where the lies end and the truth begins.' South African National Prosecuting Authority spokesman Nathi Ncube expresses disappointment with the outcome, but says the decision of the court will be respected and there will not be an appeal. He says, 'It is unfortunate that Mr Dewani has been acquitted because we believe that he was involved. The court did not find that he was innocent. The court could not rely on the evidence given by three witnesses who themselves had been convicted of the crime.' The Hindocha family say they have been failed by the justice system. Their desperate need for the truth about what happened to Anni Dewani on the night of 13 November 2010 remains unmet.

I cannot help. I don't know. I never asked Shrien Dewani whether he was involved in the murder of his wife. It was not my business. My task was to assess whether he was ill and treat him if necessary so that he could appear in court to face the charges against him. I also believe that, had I asked him, it would almost certainly have had a negative impact on whatever relationship I had with him. I did not want to jeopardise anything that might further delay his appearance in court.

To this day I feel angered and exasperated by the outcome. I think South Africa – and in particular the prosecuting authorities – shamefully failed the Hindocha family.

It is difficult for me not to feel that I also failed the family, and that the profession of psychiatry had wrongfully been involved and that the confusion of psychiatric diagnoses had complicated this tragic course of events. I believe that I am one of very many who share with the family of Anni Dewani a perception of justice having been thwarted, and an anger at the role played by psychiatry in what I believe many thought to be the obstruction of the administration of justice.

In among all the noise and clamour surrounding these events the focus seems to have become blurred or lost. A young woman was brutally murdered. A life full of hope and beauty and promise was lost. I cannot imagine what anguish this has caused the family, and must surely continue to afflict them.

28

The problem with depression

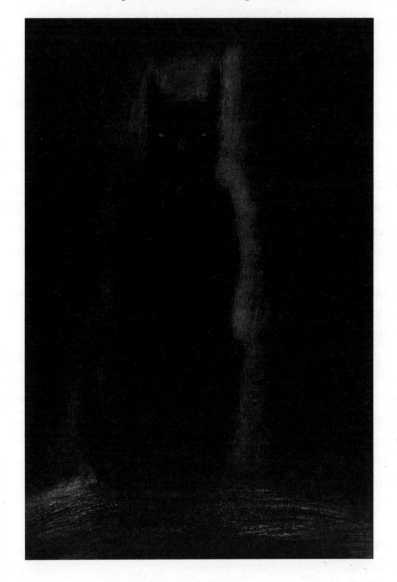

The problem with depression is, to some extent, its vocabulary. Depression is part of life. It is inevitable. In many ways it represents the burden of self-consciousness. Not to feel depressed at times is not to be quite alive, as it would be not to feel joyful or sad or apprehensive.

The difficulty arises regarding thresholds and contexts. It might be understandable, and regarded with a degree of sympathy, if at times one might become depressed while pondering the futility of life given the certainty of death. But this might also be regarded as ridiculous and self-indulgent if it persisted, to the exclusion of any other emotion that might mitigate such a gloomy appraisal and make life worth living.

Depression in the context of loss and bereavement is appropriate and necessary. It is an integral part of the process of recovery and restitution. Depression in another context, for example at a time of celebration, might be less so. A degree of depression or a sadness might not infrequently occur at the end of the day with the setting sun, and arise from a reflection on the passing of time. It would be recognised as transient and might be regarded with some indulgence, if not bemusement. Waking in the morning with sunlight bursting through the bedroom window and feeling an utter exhausting dread is altogether another matter.

Depression in the quotidian use of the word is relatively benign. In its malignant forms, it seems to be something qualitatively different. It is very often less understandable in terms of the context, and it is of a different degree and nature. It is another, different beast.

'I can't understand it,' Stefanus says. We are meeting for the first time in the outpatient clinic. He is ill-kempt and his speech is slow and monotonous. 'There is no reason for me to be this way. Nothing has gone wrong. There is no particular crisis. There is no major problem at work. There are no difficulties at home. I have a supportive wife. I am embarrassed. I feel ashamed. I just can't seem to pull myself together. I feel hopeless. I am hopeless. This has come from nowhere.'

There do not seem to be any identifiable stressors. He is a reasonably successful middle-aged businessman. Apart from raised blood pressure he is relatively healthy. The only clue is that something similar had happened to his father, who had committed suicide when Stefanus was in his late teens. 'I coped with it somehow,' he tells me in regard to this. 'I just got on with things. I have always regarded myself as a strong person. That's why I find this so difficult to cope with. It's not me.'

He describes an insidious onset. Perhaps the first indication was a difficulty in concentrating at work. Tasks that he was used to performing easily became onerous. He struggled for the first time to sleep through the night. He was finding himself waking in the early hours of the morning filled with a trepidation that he could not fathom. He had no appetite and lost a considerable amount of weight. His libido was extinguished. The worst, he says, was an overwhelming, enervating fatigue, and a profoundly distressing loss of interest and pleasure in all the things that had previously sustained him. He says there is no longer colour in his life. There is no variation in tone or pitch in the world around him. All senses are dulled. There is only a bleak and pervasive emptiness.

He had been an enthusiastic gardener but now, he says, he simply could not be bothered. His wife describes him gazing upon the ruin of the once immaculate garden with blank disinterest. When she attempts to encourage him to do some work in the garden, hoping that some simple, pleasurable task might kindle the process of recovery, his response is irritable and impatient. She simply doesn't understand, he tells her, and insists that she leave him alone. His small children are bewildered: their loving father is absent. The wife becomes angry and frightened and confused. She says she feels that there is something very wrong but has no idea what it might be or where she should turn for help. It has to be something physical, she says, to account for the extent of his decline. An assessment of depression does not make much sense to her. There is no reason for him to be depressed, she says, and anyway depression is psychological and therefore could not explain the dramatic physical deterioration that is so evident to her and to me.

Another part of the problem of depression arises from this dualist way of thinking. Depression has grave physical consequences, most obviously suicide. Defined as being psychological, in a materialist culture in particular depression is perceived to be of less import than a general medical condition. In my experience patients are acutely aware of this implicitly dismissive attitude, and this failure of understanding compounds the sense of shame and isolation and hopelessness they describe.

Consequences less dramatic than suicide are also potentially dangerous. Anthony has stopped his anti-hypertensive medication. Again, he says he couldn't be bothered. He denies suicidal intent but does say he thinks his life is not worth living. He would not mind if he had a stroke or a heart attack, or if he just happened to die. It would be some sort of solution. Perhaps it would be better for his family, a relief of the burden of having to look after him. Yes, he reflects in the presence of his appalled wife, although he is not going to kill himself – he does not have the energy, anyway – perhaps he would be better off dead.

People who are severely depressed don't look after themselves in the most basic way. They don't have the energy and they don't care. In depressed states people do not bother to exercise; they have no motivation and no energy. They do not take their medication. They smoke. They use alcohol and other drugs, either because they do not care or out of a desperate need to escape, however briefly, from the dark entrapment of their worlds.

It is understandable that one might seek escape by resorting to alcohol, an easily available and apparently extremely effective agent. Use and misuse are compounded by tolerance. More and more of the substance has to be used to achieve the same effect. A downward spiral develops into a vortex. A complex web of psychological and physical and social problems ensues, closing the trap. Social isolation, physical ailments, depression and alcohol are all risk factors for suicide, either in overt or less direct forms. Escape is no longer imagined as possible. There is no hope; the only avenue is descent into oblivion.

I tried and failed to help a colleague who was also a friend. There had been difficulties, but nothing that seemed insurmountable in the early stages. He had used alcohol for as long as I had known him, perhaps excessively but not in a way that I thought was out of control. Then he suffered what was perhaps a major disappointment in that a funding proposal was rejected. He seemed to lose direction, or make too much of this setback, and gave up seeking funding from other sources. He began to drink more heavily and his partner complained. She said he became morose and apathetic. His work performance declined and his colleagues began to express concern.

He was living in another city at the time and I went to visit him. Initially he seemed to be his old self. He expressed pleasure in seeing me and I thought and hoped that the fears had been exaggerated. He prepared a meal and suggested that we have a drink together to celebrate my visit. It felt churlish to refuse and I worried that I might alienate him. There was a fairly animated conversation at the beginning, but he was drinking steadily and then he seemed to lose concentration. It was evening and getting dark but he did not seem to register. We sat together in the gloom and his conversation became increasingly rambling and disjointed and then incoherent. I switched the lights on and he faced me in silence, immobile, as if confounded by something that he could not articulate and that had overwhelmed him. I somehow got him to bed and left the next day. A fortnight later he put a gun to his head and ended his life. We sought to console ourselves that by that stage there was nothing we could have done to stop him, but the sense of guilt and failure was inescapable. It is one of the consequences of such a malignant trajectory, the helplessness of those trying to help.

Bastiaan says he does not need help. I see him in the outpatient clinic at the request of his friends. He is HIV-positive and depressed. He has given up. He says there is nothing to live for. He has stopped eating. He does not wash himself and is refusing antiretroviral medication. He has alienated himself from his family and lost his job, and his friends have become exasperated by his apparent refusal to help himself and his rejection of hope. He dismisses the proposal of antidepressant medication, as he did the antiretrovirals. It is pointless, he says. In his way of thinking, the situation is clear and it is hopeless. It is so often a tangled, complex story, but it seems clear to us that his depression, and the decisions and the behaviour that flow from it, will eventually lead to his death. A difficult and ethically complicated aspect of the treatment of a severe depression is that the hopelessness that is part of the depression so often leads to the rejection of treatment.

Extreme forms of depression may develop a psychotic intensity. In schizophrenic states the content of delusions tends to be mystifyingly incongruent. A person might describe being pursued by unknown assailants intent on killing him or her, but appear to be nonchalant. In a severe depression a person might describe the same experience, but say the persecution is right and proper. He or she is so irredeemably bad and guilty that he or she deserves to die.

A schoolteacher I met in one of the community clinics had a vivid memory of his depression that had required an emergency admission many years previously. It was difficult for me to imagine – he seemed so well and informed and insightful. He had fully recovered and had returned to work as a secondary-school teacher. He was clearly respected by his colleagues and happily married with two teenage children. I had seen him regularly over a period of about six months and thought I had got to know him fairly well, so I suggested that he might consider a trial period without medication. He declined, saying that the memory of that depressive episode was so terrible that he did not want to put himself at any risk of a relapse. Another few months passed before he told me that he had discussed the issue with his wife and family; the decision, given the stability of his mood over the past ten years, was to embark on a cautious withdrawal. I organised a very gradual programme of reducing and stopping the medication and made an appointment to see him in a month's time. He dutifully kept the appointment but when he entered the interview room he appeared dishevelled and perplexed. Worried, I asked him how he was doing. He did not answer for a while and then whispered, 'Doctor, are you carrying a gun?' I said no, of course not, and asked why was he was asking this strange question. He said, 'I am a dog. I'm just a dirty dog and you must shoot me.'

He did recover, as he had done previously, but there was to be no further attempt at withdrawal. Sadly, it did mean that the depression was something that he was going to have to live with, that it was not some sort of aberration and that it was in some way part of him. There was to be no cure, just an acceptance – perhaps a resignation – that this malevolent dog he had momentarily become would be always lurking at the periphery of his otherwise bright life.

The problem with depression and the language used to describe its wide range of expression is also in the way it should be managed. 'Severe' and 'less severe' give some indication of a continuum, but are inadequate terms. Nevertheless, on one side of the spectrum there seems to be a syndrome more related to adverse life circumstances, and on the other a syndrome less associated with external circumstances and having more the nature of an illness. There is an apparent paradox in the way in which these two forms respond to treatment, and particularly pharmacological treatment, in that the more severe forms of depression are more responsive to treatment. It is understandable that socioeconomic ills or bereavement are unlikely to be ameliorated by a chemical agent, whereas the more severe forms of depression – which seem more probably to have a biological basis – should be more likely to respond. Treating the hardships of life with an antidepressant medication fails to acknowledge difficult and complex life circumstances, offering rather a simplistic, paternalistic, pharmacological sop, and can undermine the necessary and more constructive process of developing the resources to cope with adversity as best as possible.

What is certainly not helpful is being dismissive. This takes many forms, covert at times, and may be well intentioned. 'Don't worry, it's not so bad', 'it will be all right, it will pass with time', 'the same thing happened to me and I got over it' are likely to be heard as mere noise by a depressed person, or confirmation of a failure to understand.

Finding the right balance can be difficult. It is rarely one thing or the other; whatever form it takes, depression is a grim reality. There is a tension between acknowledging suffering and seeking to suppress its various manifestations. The woman in the clinic whose husband has been abusive and has deserted her and who now frets about how she might support her family for the month does not expect me to take her problems away. Another person, incapacitated and tormented by fatigue and a total absence of volition and afflicted with thoughts of suicide, will more probably seek any form of help – or possibly not, if in the depths of depression the situation is perceived as being beyond hope.

29

The illusory thrill of mania

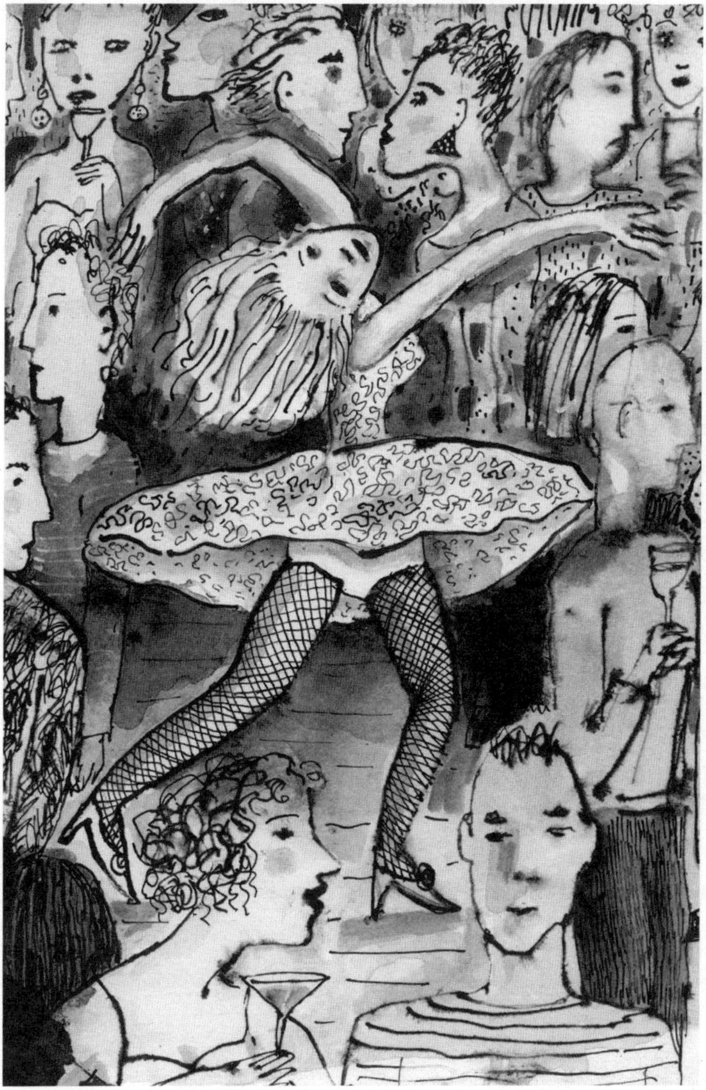

I have never encountered someone in the joyful throes of a manic state. By the time of the admission it is over. We have to cope with the aftermath, the appalled family, the shame and the anger. But even at the high pitch of the mania I am not sure of the joyfulness of it. More often our patients have described feeling out of control and being frightened. It is not an exuberant liberating epiphanous state, they say in retrospect. It is more a joyless frenzy.

Pieter sits hunched in a chair in the outpatient clinic. He was recently discharged after yet another relapse of a bipolar illness. At the time of his admission he was manic. He was not full of joy. He was not on top of the world. He was hostile, irritable and extremely aggressive. He was violent towards the nursing staff who tried to calm him. His language was abusive and obscene and racist.

I have known him for years. This is completely uncharacteristic. His manner is usually cautious and considerate. His attitude towards me seemed curiously formal at times, as if he needed to keep me at a distance. This was perhaps understandable, given that I had known a side of him that he struggled to acknowledge and which he sought to hide from the world. He had been an extremely successful businessman. It is quite possible, but merely speculative, that part of the success had owed something to an energy of incipient mania that had subsequently spun out of control.

Now everything is in ruins. He is bankrupt. His wife has left him. His friends have fled. His reputation is destroyed and in his world this also means his future. He is particularly distressed by his daughter's refusal to have any contact with him. She is angry and says she has lost all patience. Following a previous episode, he apologised to her and promised to take the medication. It came to nothing. He stopped the treatment and very soon things began to take a predictable and frightening course. He made reckless business decisions. He drank heavily and perhaps the worst for her was that he made embarrassingly inappropriate sexual advances towards her friends. She is ashamed of him. Trying to explain that this is part of an illness means little to her. He knows he has a bipolar disorder, she says. He knows what will happen when he stops the treatment. She cannot look after him. He is her father but he has failed her. She has to get on with her own life, she says, and it would be best if she now cut off all contact with him.

Sitting opposite me Pieter seems exhausted and defeated. He makes no excuse for what has happened. He does not seek to blame the illness. I ask about the future and he just heaves a weary sigh. He can see no future. This is not a depressive phase of a bipolar illness. It is the understandable and familiar aftermath of a manic episode. Given his perception of the hopelessness of the situation I am compelled to ask him about suicide. He appears to ponder this option for some time and then says no, he does not have the energy. He then says with some bitterness that it would be a solution for his business colleagues and his lost friends and family. He is trapped.

A similar tired, exasperated and angry response was described to me by the mother of Thembakosi. Again, she had been through this too many times. She had tried so hard. She had been hopeful so many times. And so many times she had had her hopes dashed. But she was his mother and she had to stay with him. There was nobody else. He had alienated all other members of his family and all his friends.

The first episode was while he was at university. He was an exceptionally bright student. In retrospect he was probably veering into mania, and it seemed that this was in part due to academic pressures – he was about to write his final exams for a degree in commerce. For no apparent reason Thembakosi assaulted a fellow student. At the time of his admission to our unit thereafter he was clearly manic, but by this time he had been expelled from the university. A tribunal was held and I managed to persuade the university authorities to allow him to write the final examinations, although he remained barred from attending lectures. He passed; everybody was happy and relieved. Whether to celebrate his success, or possibly because he could not accept the diagnosis, Thembakosi stopped the treatment and relapsed and was back in the unit within months. This sequence of events went on for years. After yet another admission he would sit facing me in the outpatient clinic and say earnestly, 'Doctor, I have learnt my lesson. I can see what damage this has done to my life and how much suffering this has caused my family. It will never happen again.' I did not doubt his determination, but it was not to be.

Months later I received a call from his mother. I am sorry, she said, as if she herself had somehow failed me. She sounded exhausted, beyond anger now, as if all her strength in keeping the family together had finally been depleted. On this occasion Thembakosi had become bored with the human resources position his father had managed to find for him. He had developed the quite brilliant notion that he could make a lot more money gambling than he could working in a job that he found unfulfilling. In one night he lost a fortune. He somehow managed to get access to his parents' credit cards and used all their money. He continues to pay off the debt. The mother said, 'He is my son. I can't turn my back on him,' but the father just stared into the distance, absent, as if there was nothing further that he could say. The family – Thembakosi, his parents, his sister, his ex-wife and their young child – seemed at that moment to be broken. Again I formed the impression that it was a great struggle for him to be well, to be a responsible son and husband and father and worker, and that at times these demands became insuperable, and like an alcoholic reaching for the next drink he succumbed to the joyless abandonment of this struggle.

These manic episodes are expressed in many different ways, and the differences between men and women are often marked. For men, aggression and violent behaviour often associated with drunkenness were common precipitants to admission to our unit. Violence provokes violence, and the effects are enduring. Enraged by his mother's entreaties to stop his excessive drinking, Kerneels in a manic fury attacked her. The father could not restrain his son. He hit him repeatedly in a desperate attempt to subdue him. We met the family after Kerneels had been admitted. They were all appalled by what had happened. This time it was not, 'This is not my son.' It was, 'This is not our family.' I think such manic episodes have a more devastating effect on families than any other form of mental illness.

Inappropriate sexual behaviour seems to be a more common expression of mania among women. A dismayed mother described her daughter's behaviour at a party hosted by her brothers. She was drinking heavily and nobody could stop her. But it was not just drunkenness, the mother said. She herself seemed reluctant to describe the events, and it was clear that the whole family had been profoundly embarrassed by the young woman's disinhibited behaviour. It was not flirtatious or amusing in any way, the mother said – it was lewd. The party had been ruined. Her dismay was compounded by her sons' subsequent refusal to have any further contact with their sister. It did not matter that she was manic, that she was ill in a way that might have been difficult for a young person to understand. They were ashamed of her.

Parties and especially wedding celebrations can be fraught affairs for people of a manic disposition. I attended the wedding of a friend whose sister was known to be struggling with a bipolar disorder. The sister began to dance wildly after the ceremony. She hauled elderly and bewildered men to their feet and frolicked about them in an increasingly hectic and lascivious manner. This being a wedding celebration, there was initially much goodwill. She was just having a good time. She was just being wild and unconventional, we wished to believe, but this gradually shifted to unease. To my dismay she then headed for me. She cavorted about me and then grabbed me towards her, pushing herself against me. 'Help me,' she whispered urgently. 'Help me. Stop me. I am out of control. You have to help me.' Perhaps at some point there was for her a blissful moment of sheer exuberance, but it was ephemeral, and my memory is of a beautiful young woman trapped in joyless agitation.

It might seem impoverished or churlish to describe the excitement of mania as illusory, given the extensive literature about the association of genius with mental illness, and mania in particular. Conventional ways of thinking and seeing and hearing are blown away by the liberating and exhilarating force of a manic episode. The corollary is that it is profoundly unimaginative – if not destructive – to attempt to control or subdue this potentially creative force. If only people with mania were allowed to roam free, unfettered by convention or medication, the world would be a brighter and more exciting place. This seems to be a romantic, wishful position, and I doubt that those suffering from bipolar disorders or their families or communities would subscribe to it. It does nevertheless seem very possible that those who have lived through these extreme states of turmoil and who have developed strategies of coping might have a wider, more imaginative sense of being in the world, and something valuable to communicate. Whether this might be considered fortunate or a blessed endowment of any kind is another matter.

Johannes said to me, 'Mania is a selfish illness. I want the mania. I miss it but I cannot cope with what it has done to my family. I cannot afford it. Not any longer.'

I have never been manic. I don't know and cannot imagine what it is like. It might then seem presumptuous to describe the possible thrill of mania as illusory. But the patients I have encountered either in the throes of mania or in its aftermath have described no joy. They have nevertheless described an intense ambivalence about both the nature of the experience and how it should be managed. For the most part it is accepted that it is not possible to live this way. But with this acceptance something is lost. Something is sacrificed. Treatment represents some form of compromise, as if some important part of oneself is being suppressed. Achieving the balance of holding the energy, the exhilarating sense that all things are possible, and preventing the ensuing chaos and disorganisation is exasperatingly difficult and elusive.

30

The allure of intoxication

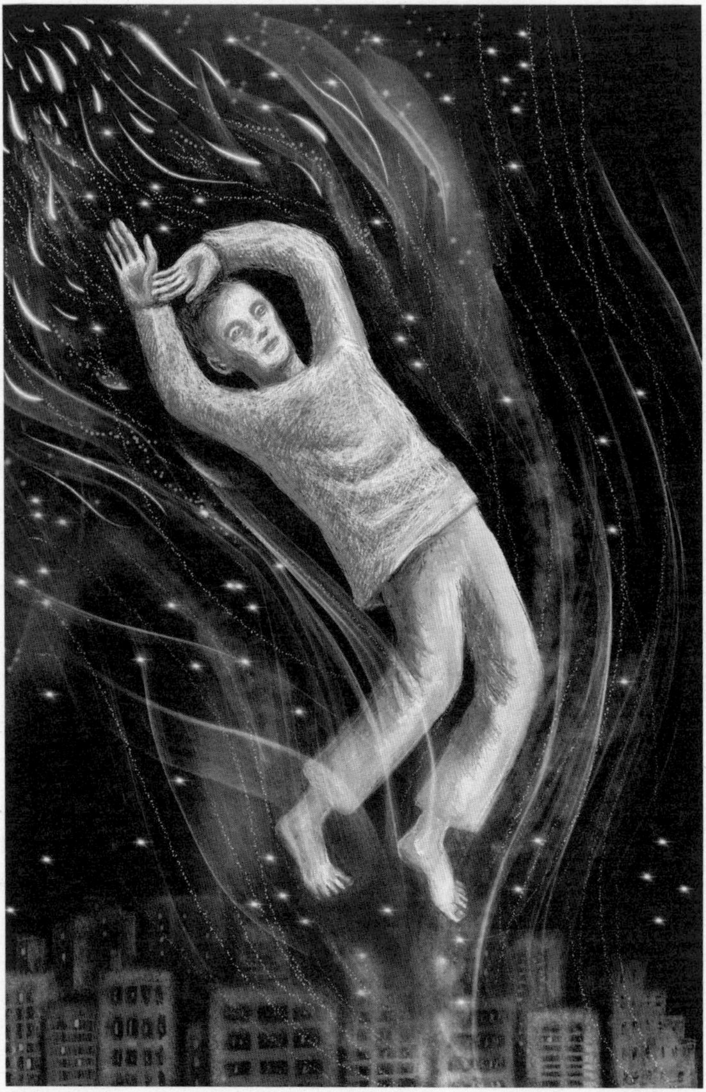

'I don't understand it. How could you do this? How could you do this to your family? How could you do this to yourself? I don't know what to say. Honestly, I don't know what to do. I'm finished.'

The mother sighs and stares ahead, angry, looking at nothing.

Xolisi slumps in his chair, his legs splayed, his eyes downcast in a posture of defiant nonchalance. The occupational therapist fidgets and stifles a yawn. The students look away from mother and son, embarrassed by the mother's distress. The silence is oppressive. There is nothing I can say to console her or to reassure her. I think it is important that she speaks and that we listen, but I am not sure that it will help her and I am a little bit more sure that it is not going to make any difference. This has happened before and it is going to happen again. Xolisi will get better. We will discharge him and within a few months he will be back and we will listen again to the mother vent her fury and exasperation.

She has to deal with this on her own. The father is absent. The community has shunned her. When intoxicated Xolisi has been violent and stolen from the neighbours to obtain the drugs he uses that make him mad. The mother's anger is compounded by shame. To add to her woes she is poverty-stricken. Xolisi is her only child. He is unemployable. She asks whether at least she can apply for a disability grant. The social worker is stern. Xolisi is not sick or disabled, she says, in that he brings this problem on himself. If he did not use the drugs, he could go out and find work. He must take responsibility. He does not qualify for a disability grant. The mother sighs, defeated. I turn to Xolisi, attempting to prompt a response. He refuses. He has also heard this all before. He has been through this time and time again and he is telling us that there is nothing for him to say. The occupational therapist excuses herself. She says she has another meeting to attend but I think she is bored. If it is not Xolisi, it is Thabo or Jan or Yusuf. It's the same old sad, predictable story. We are going around in circles.

It is a struggle not to become resigned or angry, to imagine Xolisi not as just another member of a lost and aimless tribe of young and hopeless men. I try to imagine him, crouched in some dark and empty space, the wind tearing at the frail corrugated-iron shelter, the loneliness, the menace of poverty and deprivation outside, craving that moment of bliss, that rapturous escape, the lighting of the pipe, the rattle of the crystals against the glass, the luxurious inhalation of the fumes that are familiar but also thrilling. He is transformed. Nothing matters, not for this wonderful moment when he can imagine he can do anything, that things are not as they are and that he is free.

Intoxication is not a form of madness. It is a transient, self-limiting phenomenon arising from the effects of whichever psychoactive substance has been used. These effects are broadly categorised as being stimulant or depressant or hallucinogenic in the derangement of perceptions. The euphoria sometimes associated with alcohol use is due to the depressant action on the higher inhibitory centres of the brain. There seems to be something sad in the observation that the most evolved and highly developed parts of ourselves are negative or inhibitory, in limiting ourselves, and it is perhaps a factor in our persisting use of a drug that is so obviously harmful. We imagine, in a state of happy intoxication, that we are more ourselves.

Intoxicated people do not come to our unit. If there is extremely disturbed behaviour, they might be admitted to a casualty unit where they cause much havoc and anger among the nursing and medical staff. This is not uncommon, particularly over the weekends; it is potentially dangerous and it is complicated. The danger of course can be due to the drunken disruption of emergency care, but it can also be due to less obvious causes. We cannot assume that the disorganised behaviour is due solely to intoxication. When they are drunk and disinhibited people do stupid and dangerous things. They fight and fall over. The casualty staff, very often harassed and overworked in the chaos of medical and surgical emergencies, therefore have to be alert for the potentially lethal effects of head injuries. These injuries might not be immediately obvious. A closed head injury might have no external sign. An assumption might very easily be made that the altered level of consciousness is due to intoxication and hours later the person is found dead due to a rupture of a blood vessel within the brain.

The situation can also be complicated in that it might not be straightforward, clinically, to distinguish an intoxicated state from a psychosis. A psychosis implies a clear consciousness, differentiating it from delirium. But defining and identifying an altered level of consciousness is fraught with difficulty. Broadly, and perhaps rather simplistically, clear consciousness may be inferred by the ability to focus, sustain and shift attention appropriately. This can be very difficult to determine in a person in a floridly psychotic state. Psychosis does not protect against intoxication. On the contrary, it seemed very often that our patients intoxicated themselves to escape the burden of their psychoses.

The matter is further complicated by the fact that intoxication might induce a psychosis. In this circumstance, the intoxicated state is not limited to the time in which the psychoactive substance exerts its effects on the brain, but shades into a persistent psychosis independent of the direct effects of the substance. This is perhaps most marked with regard to cannabis or dagga. It is this induced psychosis that brings Xolisi back to our unit time and time again.

Exposure to cannabis increases the risk of developing a psychosis, more specifically schizophrenia, two- to threefold. The increased risk is associated with the amount of exposure and the concentration of the psychoactive ingredients, and exposure is particularly hazardous before the age of approximately fifteen. At this stage the brain undergoes a number of subtle and complex changes – including a process described as synaptic pruning whereby unnecessary or unused neuronal connections are discarded or edited out. This is also the stage when young people are most likely to start using cannabis, if only in the spirit of experimentation. The theory is that it is this disorganisation of neuronal connections – owing to a genetic vulnerability and environmental factors including exposure to cannabis – that form the neurobiological basis of schizophrenia. It is therefore quite mad – or it constitutes a high risk – if having a family history of schizophrenia one voluntarily exposes oneself at a young age to cannabis. Yet this happened all too frequently in our unit, and it seemed all the more tragic arising out of ignorance or a false and romantic notion of the innocuous allure of intoxication.

Another hazardous consequence of this allure is of course addiction. One can be intoxicated without becoming addicted and one can be addicted to a substance without being intoxicated. Some of the elements of the clinical syndrome of addiction include a feeling of compulsion to use the substance despite its harmful consequences, a priority accorded to the use, a stereotyped or routine pattern of use, withdrawal symptoms, and the phenomenon of tolerance, with more and more of the substance being required to gain the same effect.

A disease or medical or biological model has been proposed to account for the sometimes mystifying, self-destructive phenomenon of addiction. According to this way of thinking, the problem arises from a distortion or derangement of the natural and fundamental processes that ensure survival. Eating and drinking and sexual activity are associated with pleasurable feelings or rewards that encourage the repetition of these behaviours, which in turn enable us to continue living and encourage procreation. The allure of intoxication and the associated problem of addiction provide a false reward that does not ensure health and survival.

There seems to be something simplistic or reductive in this, certainly if it excludes any form of personal agency or responsibility. Being adult or responsible or behaving in a civilised manner, however vague or problematic these constructs might be, includes some sense of being able to inhibit through the higher centres of the central nervous system impulses that arise in the lower centres. As much as we might need to eat and drink and have sex to live and ensure the survival of our species, we also need to control these impulses according to the context in which these activities might occur. What might be healthy and gratifying in one circumstance might be shameful and grotesquely inappropriate, if not criminal, in another.

Given some of the uncertainties regarding the notion of free will, and with it a problematic doubt regarding personal responsibility, in our daily lives there needs to be at least some sense that we have a degree of control. Eating can be a pleasurable activity, but we do not gorge ourselves to death. Sexual activity can be joyful and enhance life, but to claim an addiction to sex seems more probably a cynical manoeuvre to avoid responsibility for one's actions. To pathologise this behaviour, to invoke the concept of a disease, is to exempt the individual from responsibility. This has grave personal but also social consequences. It would surely be regarded as preposterous for a person accused of rape to seek exoneration on the basis that he had no control over his actions owing to a problem of addiction to sex. There is little doubt that addiction to alcohol has a familial or genetic predisposition, but that is what it is, a biological vulnerability rather than a genetic determination or fate. Addiction to alcohol and other substances such as the opioids is a tragic condition, and trying to make sense of it in order to be helpful is not promoted by simplistic models or facile solutions. The medical model in its reductive form is inadequate, as would be any alternative model that failed to take into account the physical components of this extremely complex phenomenon.

Some years ago, while recovering from a serious back operation, I was prescribed morphine. This had a most memorable and blissful effect. I think it was on the fifth day after the surgery that I recall having to make a very conscious and determined effort not to request any further doses of the opioid. A degree of pain was preferable to what seemed to me a very real possibility of becoming addicted. As has been described so often, it was not so much that the pain was dramatically diminished but that it did not matter very much. It also seemed possible that this mysterious nonchalance could have been extended to the problem of addiction, that it might not matter too much as long as I was guaranteed a regular supply of the morphine.

At the time of writing it is estimated that in the USA more than thirty thousand people are dying every year due to opioid addiction. I don't know which factors stopped me from demanding more morphine in the days following the surgery, but some part of it must surely have been an understanding of the grave consequences of this apparently simple and apparently harmless act. Far too many are less fortunate.

The allure is powerful and its nature is complex. Many social and economic and psychological factors must surely contribute, and it would be inappropriate to generalise from one particular story. There does seem to be a degree of ambivalence nonetheless, or even a paradox in many of the events we encountered in our unit. In one respect it seemed that the allure of intoxication and its extension into madness was that things then did not matter too much, that the burden of consciousness was diminished. Given the dire circumstances in which many of our patients lived, this altered state was likely to be extremely seductive. In another – contrary – respect, the allure seemed to arise from a sense that it made our patients feel more like themselves, that this intoxicated and mad self was the true self, unfettered, unconfined by social constraints or by medication, liberated and intoxicated by the illusory belief that the world was a better and brighter place.

We say goodbye to Xolisi on a Friday afternoon. His mother has come to collect him. He makes a little speech. He thanks us for helping him and says that he is now well and that he feels strong enough to face the challenges that he knows await him beyond the hospital walls. He says that he has learnt an important lesson, and that he will never use drugs again. I do not doubt that Xolisi is sincere in this, and that he is determined to stop the drugs and never return to our hospital. I also do not doubt that he will return, and that we will again sit down together, his mother angry and dejected, Xolisi dumbfounded, and our staff trying against the odds to maintain, yet again, some frail hope.

31

Madness as a disorder of consciousness

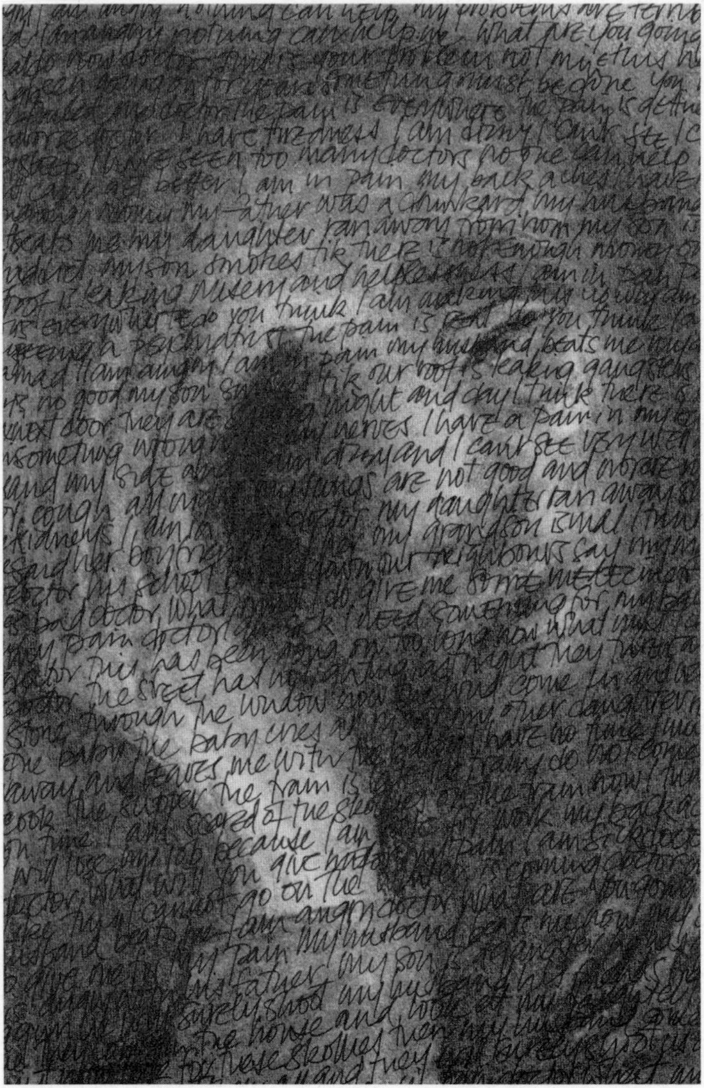

'They know what I am thinking … it is horrible … they know everything about me … how can I protect myself?' – Damian

'I am not ill … it's just a phase I am going through … the doctors stole my organs for black magic … I need a herbalist to clean my blood, not a doctor … I am working with the devil … I see the visible souls … they just stand and watch me … I have to kill myself because I am too afraid … I am fighting to take control of my mind.' – Hoosain

'You are absolutely under control … if you don't cooperate it's hell … I have no privacy … I couldn't take it.' – Arnoldus, following a suicide attempt

Although these utterances are in some ways disorganised and inconsistent, there are – in addition to the anguish – certain shared themes. There is a loss of autonomy, or the sense of being in control. The feeling of the self as being differentiated from the external world and being able to act on the world appears to have become profoundly disrupted. Definitions of consciousness are various and problematic, but generally include, at least in part, the intactness of these faculties, and it is in this respect that madness – or, more specifically, the psychoses – may be considered a disorder of a particularly human consciousness.

There is a loss of privacy, of the self being separate and therefore protected from the external world. It is described as being terrifying to the extent that suicide is considered as an escape. I am told it is a kind of hell. Things happen that should not happen in a familiar and customary world or in a shared reality. One's most vital functions, of breathing and of the heart beating, are under external and absolute command. There seems to be a losing battle for control of the mind, and in this a part of the horror must be the exquisite and paradoxical consciousness of the disorder of consciousness – of being mindful of losing one's mind.

Part of the problem of consciousness is that it may be conceptualised at different levels and that at the more basic levels its functions are clearer than at the higher levels. I need to be aware of hunger to eat to sustain myself. I need to be conscious of danger to decide whether to flee or fight. I also need to have some sense of agency, or a capacity to act on the world, to keep myself alive. These are not particularly human faculties, and consciousness in this respect is fairly simply an evolved capacity to increase ones chances of survival. A higher, more human consciousness is certainly more complex.

There is a certain poignancy in that the purpose of what might be considered our greatest endowment, our essentially human consciousness, is not at all clear to us. We do not need this higher-level consciousness to stay alive. It enables us to seek meaning, or to contemplate the possibility of meaninglessness, or of God, and to acquire knowledge, but that does not make us stronger or better or live much longer or transcend our mortality. On the contrary, human consciousness can at times seem burdensome. Much time and effort are expended in either altering or subduing our consciousness with alcohol or in other forms of intoxication, or we might seek to annihilate it altogether in acts of suicide.

If a higher-level, particularly human, reflective self-consciousness is difficult to define, and its function in the grand scheme of things is obscure, how it might arise from mere matter is yet another enigma. Some argue that having to use our consciousness to explain our consciousness makes the problem intractable. Others propose that we simply do not and will never have the capacity, being human, to make sense of it. Others consider that it is merely a matter of time, that it is a problem that can be solved – much like the nature of life on earth or the origins of the universe. The argument is not that these mysteries might drive us mad, but that it is these elusive and human qualities that become deranged in psychotic states.

I ask my patients when they are recovering and regaining a degree of insight what they think might have gone wrong, what might have caused them to become mad. Perhaps the most frequent response is, 'I think too much.' Consciousness is perceived as a burden that can become intolerable. Something that is quite enormous and grants us the dignity of our humanity has been gained, but with a loss. Being self-aware, conscious of ourselves as separate from the world, has enabled us to acquire a vast amount of knowledge and gain mastery to a great extent of our circumstances. That this might lead to eventual self-destruction is not of immediate concern. But having taken that fateful step, in Adam's making the choice to accept the apple from Eve and with it the capacity for knowledge and self-consciousness, we became banished from the Garden of Eden. We lost our innocence. In becoming aware of ourselves, we gained the capacity for shame. We lost forever the capacity for a voluptuous immersion in the oneness of the world, for many quite possibly a desirable unconsciousness, a deep and tranquil sleep, or the solace of not knowing. That is what I think my patients are telling me: 'It is all too much. My consciousness is too much for me.'

A loss of insight is a core feature of psychosis. Psychotic states might then be interpreted as a shutting down of insight into our separateness, or a refusal of consciousness. This combination of an intense self-awareness and the conviction that one is not in control is a cruel anomaly of the psychoses, and of schizophrenia in particular. I am agonisingly aware that I am not separate from the world, that I am no longer I.

Mpho says he wants or needs a circumcision. He tells us that he is not interested in whether this is done in a cultural way, with all the attendant rituals. He is determinedly pragmatic. He needs the circumcision to give him the strength to kill his enemies who are tormenting him. He is being mutilated. His brain is being devoured by dogs that are set upon him by his persecutors across the river. The only way for him to survive is for him to gain the strength to destroy his enemies in return. He is desperate and alone. He is at the mercy of his tormentors with their devouring dogs. He is terrifyingly conscious of his predicament but this consciousness does not help him to resolve the crisis. He cannot help himself. He is afflicted with the awareness of his helplessness and desperately seeks our assistance in organising the circumcision he insists he needs. He says nobody can understand what he is going through – and of course he is right.

To describe what he might be experiencing as persecutory delusions, although valid in one sense, seems pitifully inadequate. The objectively identified psychopathology is in a profoundly different realm from the felt horror of believing that your brain is being devoured by dogs. Consciousness is inherently subjective – and in that respect private and inaccessible and in some essential way unknowable. I can only with difficulty imagine what it must be like to have my brain eaten by dogs, but I can't really. It cannot even be a faint approximation. We are in two separate worlds, and this is what Mpho bewails. Nobody can possibly understand. If only this minor procedure of removing the foreskin from his penis could be performed he could begin to sort out his problems himself. He is tormented and estranged from others and the sense of a shared world by the mystifying contents of his disturbed consciousness.

Somewhere along the way this has to be dealt with, but in the midst of the crisis the first priority is to get him out of this horrifying space, to create some distance between him and the dogs. I don't think it would be very helpful to him to engage at this point in some form of psychotherapy about what it might feel like to have your brain devoured by dogs. One can only begin to imagine that it is horrifying. Pity is not going to stop it.

Bernard is bright and articulate and indignant. He is under the control of an artificial intelligence device that in turn is controlled by the ANC in collaboration with international intelligence agencies including the FBI. This conspiracy against him has developed because of his work as a developmental officer for the DA, the opposition party to the ANC. The device that has been installed in his brain controls every function, including the most intimate and private. It forces him to have erections and to masturbate in public. This is intolerable and profoundly humiliating for him and he has been admitted to our unit following a suicide attempt.

An integral component of consciousness is a sense of autonomy and free will, or at least the feeling that one is free to choose how one might act. The distinction is pertinent in the light of evidence casting some doubt on whether this might be an illusion. Based initially on electrophysiological studies, signals of brain activity are observable prior to the conscious decision to perform a simple action. This has been interpreted in many ways and does raise interesting questions about the freedom of will – and hence the nature of consciousness, and what it might mean to be human. Whether we are free in this empirical, objective sense does not detract from the feeling of being free to choose how to act in one way or another, or to choose to act or not to act.

There appears to be an unbridgeable gap between the observable, implacable world of objects and our essentially subjective world, however unknowable to others, that grants us the sense of who we are. Being intractably private makes this sense or this feeling or belief no less real, and it is the invasion of this privacy that seems so often to drive suicidal behaviour. It is a grim existential quandary in schizophrenia that, in the loss of control and autonomy, the perceived recourse of regaining control is self-destruction.

The clinical features of the schizophrenia spectrum are various but share certain core characteristics. The content of delusions or false beliefs often concerns notions of thought insertion or withdrawal, or of thought broadcasting – the feeling that one's thoughts are known to others. These clusters of symptoms are described as passivity phenomena, and are considered to be of first-rank significance in making a diagnosis of schizophrenia. These delusions are associated with various forms of thought disorder that may be described broadly as a loss of the effectiveness of one's utterances, a loss of awareness of that loss, and auditory hallucinations, a misattribution of events generated internally to the external world. The more negative cluster of symptoms, described in this way because they represent absences or deficits, are a loss of volition or a drive to action, a restricted emotional range and responsiveness, and social withdrawal. Together, these apparently disparate features share core elements in the loss of a sense of self, of the unity of the self, and of the self being autonomous. If this subjective sense of self is a core feature of a consciousness, the schizophrenias represent a profound disruption of whatever might be construed as the faculty of human self-consciousness, or who we are in the world.

Another feature of this higher-level, possibly rather vague notion of human consciousness is a sense of unity, both in the moment and over time, and of the awareness of the outside world that is personal and individual, to the extent that there is an 'I' that is the subject and at the centre of this experience. We presume ourselves to be the lead actors in our constructions and productions. This unity, or the feeling of it, becomes threatened or disorganised in psychosis. 'They know what I am thinking, it's horrible ... how can I protect myself?' is an utterance characteristic of the more positive side of the spectrum, in contrast to the confounded, catatonic states on the negative side, in which any sense of self or self-consciousness seems to have been obliterated.

Carel says nothing. He gazes through me. He is not present. It is profoundly disconcerting. I don't know where to begin. It seems impossible that we will ever retrieve him. He is lost to himself, to us, and to his family and to the world. Whatever consciousness there might be of himself and everything that surrounds him is to us a baffling mystery.

The lamentation 'I think too much' raises the question whether the disorder of consciousness is not a deficit but an excess of consciousness, a loss of balance and filter and proportion with the result that one becomes overwhelmed and engulfed by the world.

In the seventeenth century Descartes proposed 'I think therefore I am', arguing for reason or thinking as a defining characteristic of human consciousness. My patients were telling me, 'I think too much, therefore I am lost to who I am.' There is a neurobiological correlate to this. Too much thinking might be interpreted as corresponding to too much connectivity in the brain. In late adolescence synaptic pruning takes place. This editing or refining developmental process should enable us to become more efficient, to focus attention, to develop the capacity for judgement and to plan and problem-solve, the very faculties that become impaired in schizophrenia. It seems that this enormously complex and delicate process becomes disorganised in schizophrenia, presumably as a consequence of an interplay of genetic and environmental factors, and the stage of life at which this occurs corresponds frequently to the time of onset of schizophrenia. Through the loss of an effective filtering, there is a surfeit of redundant connections leading to a storm of signals to the higher centres. We are incapacitated; attaching meaning or attributing salience is random and all becomes noise.

We have much to learn from madness about the nature of human consciousness.

It is a curious paradox that schizophrenia might be imagined as a condition of being both less or too much of whomever we might be. An intricate balance is lost.

32

Madness as a disorder of self

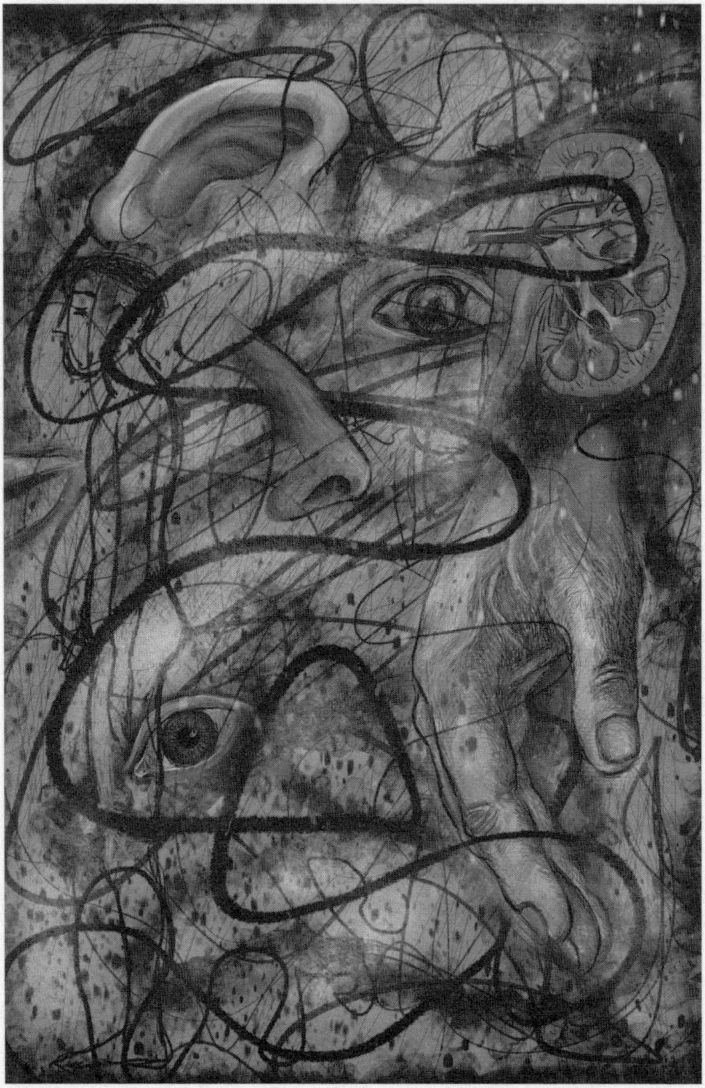

'No, that is not me. It's been put there.'

'What do you mean?'

'I don't know. Maybe it was some sort of transplant.'

'Are you telling us that your face, your nose, your mouth, your ears, that this has all been transplanted?'

'Yes, I think so. Maybe.'

'Your eyes?'

'Yes, my eyes also. All of it.'

'What do you mean, all of it?'

'Everything. Me.'

'Your skin? Your whole body? Your brain?'

'Yes. But not all at the same time. It just happened.'

'But then if everything, absolutely everything, has been transplanted in some way, who are you?'

Hoosain gazes vaguely around the room. He seems bemused by the question, as if it is of no consequence.

He shrugs.

'I don't know.' And then, as an afterthought, 'It doesn't matter.'

His posture is one of indifference. His tone of voice is flat, on the edge of irritation at my persistent questioning regarding a matter he seems to consider trite and irrelevant.

Perhaps this is what many of us in the room find disconcerting. His apparent nonchalance challenges our assumptions of the notion of the self, of the unity of the self and the notion of the self being dear to us. There might at times be conflict, we might on occasion be angry or ashamed of ourselves and particularly in adolescence we might wish that we were not ourselves, but it is profoundly curious to disown oneself. To do so in such an emphatic way, to insist that one is not oneself, both in a physical and a psychological sense, is not merely a bizarre impossibility but compels an anxious questioning about our own confidence in the privacy and unity of the self.

Hoosain addresses a curious predicament. He is not himself, and yet he is embodied. The evidence of his physical being is clear to everybody in the room. In an attempt to resolve this apparent contradiction he has constructed an elaborate and very strange explanation – that he has been transplanted – except that he quite obviously does not think it is strange. It is nevertheless some sort of answer, because although it is not himself, something resembling himself is evidently there.

Hoosain was brought to the community clinic by his anxious family and then referred to our unit. It is perhaps an unusual story in that in this instance there is no dramatic event that precipitated the admission. There has been no crazed behaviour, no violence. He is a bright, devout and caring young man, but in the few months before he came to us he has drifted away, his mother says. He is not himself. He is elsewhere. His family is dismayed and mystified. He is described as a rather placid, unassuming young man. He has recently completed his schooling, and if there is a stressful circumstance his mother wonders whether it might be due to some uncertainty about what direction he might take in life. This is speculative. He has never expressed any concerns to her. He is a private young man and she thinks it best to respect this privacy. Now she is angry and frightened. Her son is denying and disowning himself, and in this way his mother and his family.

'What has happened, Doctor? Is it me? Is it something I have done? This is not my son. Bring him back to me. My son is sick. You must bring him back to our family.'

I don't think the word 'schizophrenia' means anything to her, or provides any meaningful explanation for the devastating changes that have taken place in her absent yet present son. Yet one way of understanding schizophrenia – or, more specifically, the psychopathology or the experience of schizophrenia – is to imagine it as a disorder of the self or of self-consciousness. The notion of self is fluid and various across time and culture, but broadly includes in some way the concepts of unity, privacy and autonomy, or some belief at least that we might be in control of our thoughts and actions. It is these very feelings or beliefs or assumptions that become disorganised in schizophrenia. One is no longer in control of one's thoughts. There is a machine manipulated by alien and persecutory forces that control every thought and action. There is no privacy. Thoughts are broadcast to all and sundry. Although my thinking and my mood and behaviour might change to some extent over time and in different situations, I have a fundamental sense of a self that is continuous and unitary. I am my own, until such time that I might become afflicted with such a profoundly dreaded altered state of being.

Hoosain has lost all that. He is dispersed, fragmented, arbitrarily and ineffectually reconstituted in random bits and pieces. He is also broken in another way. There is no correspondence or unity of thinking and feeling. If I were to believe that somebody had stolen my thoughts I would be very angry. If I were to conclude that my friends were my enemies and hell-bent on trying to kill me I would be very distressed and very frightened. Hoosain is neither angry nor afraid. He seems blank, perhaps (although I am not sure if this is my own imputation) baffled by the extraordinary events that have overtaken him.

Given the depth and pervasiveness of these deranged states it is difficult to imagine how we could possibly hope to put him back together again.

Sometimes I have found myself dreaming whimsically of being an orthopaedic surgeon. A simple X-ray could identify the broken part. A relatively simple procedure could reset the fracture and the problem would be solved. Of course nothing is that simple but in this domain of psychosis we do not even understand clearly what is broken in order to fix it. It is difficult, or it seems utterly inadequate, to attribute these profoundly disturbing experiences of a disordered self to a dysregulation of dopamine transmission or any other neurobiological fault.

Perhaps the high value attached to the self in the frenzied narcissism of the present day is unusual, and amplified by social media and other technological advances. The extent to which this might translate into a greater sense of confidence in the self or in the sense of being in control of one's circumstances is unclear. A paradox seems to have arisen in that the high accord attached to the self appears to be associated with an increase in misery and insecurity, if the relatively recent increase in self-harm, depression and suicide among young people may be considered indicators of this disturbing trend. We do not so happily put ourselves on display. We gaze upon the enviable ways in which others present themselves and wonder and worry how we could possibly compete. A false virtual world holds us in thrall. The self presented to this ephemeral community becomes increasingly fictional; it seems plausible that a disjunction between whatever might be regarded as the true or authentic self and the virtual self is a part of this distress. Possibly imagined as self-affirming, this grim charade appears to have the opposite effect, certainly among the vulnerable, and vulnerability and a lack of self-confidence may be regarded almost as defining characteristics of young adolescents, those most engaged in the tangled webs of social media.

Ambivalence about the value or the priority accorded to the self is evident in other domains. We seek to lose ourselves in dance or meditation. We abandon ourselves in the hopeful bliss of sexual intimacy. We unburden ourselves of the consciousness of ourselves in alcohol and the misuse of other psychoactive substances. We aspire to transcend ourselves in the worship of the divine, and most definitively and tragically we destroy ourselves in acts of suicide. It does not seem to be without question that we regard our self-consciousness as an unreserved blessing.

The value attached to the self in relation to the community has some pertinence to varying outcomes in schizophrenia across cultures. Rather unexpectedly, given limited resources, outcomes in developing countries have been shown in some studies to be superior to those in developed, better-resourced countries. There are a number of possible explanations for these anomalous findings. It is conceivable that in highly individualistic, materialistic societies a person disabled by mental illness would be ostracised as worthless because he or she is unproductive. Conversely, in a less formal economy someone living with a serious mental illness might be accorded a degree of dignity in performing unskilled but valued work, for example taking care of young children in an extended family.

Another possible factor is that psychotic symptoms in traditional contexts may be granted meaning and are therefore socially and culturally validated. Hearing voices might be interpreted as receiving messages from the ancestors. The person is then more likely to be granted a certain status and included in the community, rather than being excluded and alienated for demonstrating symptoms of madness. Another factor might be the importance attached to the self in western cultures, in that the breakdown of the self in psychotic states might be expected to have a more devastating impact than in more communalist societies characterised by greater value being invested in the community than the individual.

I have observed these differences in our hospital. Among the more advantaged families, and this often but not always correlates with being white, there seems to be an extra burden of disgrace. This is deeply felt by our patients of course. Perhaps there is a greater degree of indignation and injustice. How could this happen to us? How could it be that our relative good fortune, our material wealth, our caring and conventional middle-class world has not provided an adequate bulwark against this strange illness? Implicit in this is a perhaps understandable need for some sort of explanation. This takes many forms, but often it is that something or someone is at fault – that there has been some sort of moral failing, and this madness is the consequence. The troubled self is further burdened with shame and guilt.

That the self is private and unique is a tenuous assumption. If grand socioeconomic and political polarities have any validity, in the capitalist, supposedly individualistic west, mass marketing seeks to impose a uniformity of need. We are persuaded that we need the newest car or the smartest smartphone to define our worth. We happily 'share' our private worlds with strangers on the internet. In one of the few countries in the world still prepared to call itself communist, a 'social credit system' is proposed. Big-data systems are to be deployed to reward citizens who are deemed to be good because they are loyal and obedient party members or patriots, and to punish those who might be of unsound political persuasions. Rewards might take the form of employment opportunities or better access to services. Punishment, because the rating and rankings are to be made public, is likely to be social exclusion. Worth is defined not as being a good consumer but as being a good citizen. On opposite sides of the world, in two opposing social and political systems, the notion of the self as private and having some sort of agency and value is undermined or abolished – and that of course has nothing to do with schizophrenia.

'You should not be ashamed of being a homosexual. Everybody is talking about it. They know what you are because of the way you talk and the way you walk. You should just accept it.'

I am taken aback, as are the students who are with me in the cramped interview room of the outpatient clinic. Jacob appears to be admonishing me.

'You were always the odd one out at school. Everybody seemed to know what was going on, except you. He said he didn't care but you know he was hurting. I said it was nobody's business but you begged to differ. You said it was wrong. I said I didn't think so but she was laughing behind your back. You see.'

He pauses and stares at me meaningfully, as if seeking confirmation that I can indeed see, but I can't. I am struggling to make sense of his utterances. One of the young medical students is attempting to stifle laughter. The consultant is being accused by his patient of being a repressed homosexual. Jacob stares at me impatiently, then embarks on a further tirade of confused sexuality, innuendo and fragmented but vivid memories. I feel myself being swept up in the current of this, trying to hold on in the turbulence to at least something that might make sense.

It then occurs to me that the problem is his random use of the personal pronoun. 'I', 'you', 'he' and 'she' are being used interchangeably. He is not referring to me but himself when he says that one should not be ashamed of one's sexuality. He is showing features of a formal thought disorder characteristic of schizophrenia – but perhaps of greater significance is the particular nature of that disorder. His shifting use of the personal pronoun seems to be an expression of his shifting sense of self. His self is disorganised. There is no stable 'I'. He is floundering, being buffeted by random events. As in an Escher etching, he is going up stairs that were going down, looking out of a window at an image of himself looking back at himself. All is to and fro and inside out and up and down. It is exhausting just listening to him, just trying to understand. I cannot imagine what it must be like for him, being on the inside.

Jacob's illness is intractable. Over the many years I've known him there has been no significant change. His curious thought disorder persists. At least now I begin to understand what might be underpinning it, although I can't imagine that makes much difference to him.

We manage to put Hoosain back together again. It seems deeply mysterious that through the manipulation of a few neurotransmitters his body can be restored to itself.

I ask him before the discharge what he makes of it, how every part of himself could have been transplanted and re-implanted. He laughs and says he must have been mad. He doesn't attend the follow-up appointment. I don't know what happens to him and can only hope that he remains intact.

33

Bring back my son

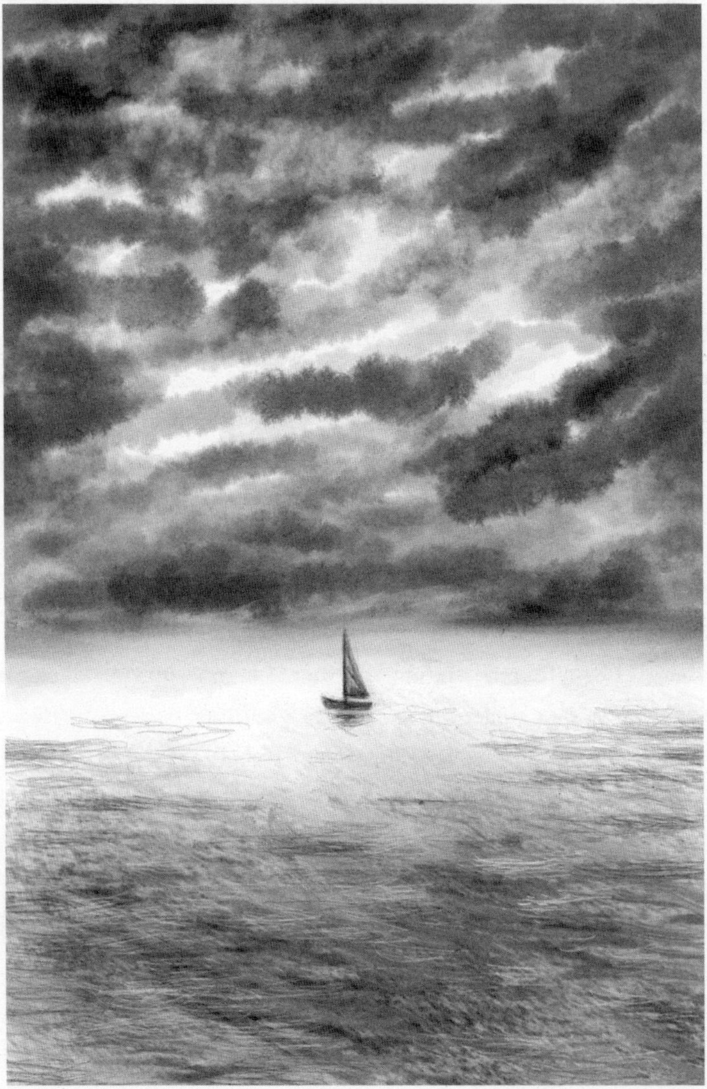

To be hopeful is fundamental to living and coping with schizophrenia, but very often this is a struggle in itself. To be hopeful is something we need to say and also to believe, but on many occasions the words have seemed hollow to me, utterances of blind faith. I listen to myself insisting to a weary family that there must always be hope, that the very uncertainty of the course of schizophrenia gives some cause for hope, and I sense their tired disbelief and resignation. But giving up hope is untenable.

There is a dismally familiar trajectory culminating in the plea, 'Doctor, bring back my son,' bring back my husband, my wife, my daughter, bring back that person I care for and who now seems so far away and so changed.

Jannes was a bright, good-looking, confident young man. There was no sign of what was to happen. There was no family history of mental illness. There were no problems at birth and no delay in the developmental milestones. He grew up in a happy, secure and stable household. He flourished at school and enjoyed playing rugby and cricket. Tentatively his parents began to entertain high hopes for his future.

Even in retrospect it is difficult to identify the point at which things began to fall apart. In his middle teens he began occasionally to use drugs. Initially this caused no great alarm. His parents reflected that this is what young people did. He was exploring, and in any event it was only cannabis, nothing dangerous like heroin. Everybody was doing it. It was an adolescent rite of passage.

But gradually he became withdrawn. He no longer seemed to care about his appearance. He seemed to be less self-assured. Previously of a cheerful disposition, he became cautious, wary, sullen. His increasingly troubled parents attributed this to adolescence. Other parents described the same behaviours in their children. Jannes drifted away. He stopped playing sport. His teachers reported that his schoolwork had begun to deteriorate. His parents confronted him. 'What is going on? What is the matter? Talk to us.'

'There is nothing wrong with me. Leave me alone,' he retorted, irritable, almost hostile. He spent increasing amounts of time locked in his bedroom. He stopped attending school. His parents did not believe that at this stage he was using drugs and so could no longer attribute this to his frightening decline. The situation deteriorated. He hardly spoke to his parents or to his younger sister. When he did he seemed vague, distant. He did not wash. The situation was becoming intolerable.

Eventually one fateful evening the parents and the daughter were uneasily having a meal. Jannes had retreated to his room. They heard a scream and the sound of breaking glass. Rushing into the room they found their son, cowering in a corner, covered in blood from a shattered mirror. He appeared to be terrified. He said it was the voices, the incessant voices, that were tormenting him and the cameras in the mirror that were monitoring his every movement. His distraught parents attempted to calm him. They managed to get him to the casualty unit of the local hospital. The harried casualty officer asked about drugs. The parents confirmed that he had used but they thought that was something of the past. The doctor concluded that parents of adolescent children often did not know what they were up to and attributed the psychotic episode to substance abuse. He prescribed benzodiazepines and sent the family home. For a short while there was an awkward calm. The medication made him tranquil, but he seemed to have lost all spontaneity. He was distracted, remote. The family struggled on.

It was only after a further dramatic event that he was admitted to our unit. He had again withdrawn to his room. His mother, hovering anxiously outside the door, listened to him muttering and cursing. She forced her way into the room and shouted at him: 'What is the matter with you?'

'The voices, the voices!' he screamed. 'It's the cameras. Don't you understand? Don't you people know what's going on?'

'That's nonsense, you are talking nonsense. You are sick,' she countered, terrified and exhausted. He lunged at her, his hands about her throat. Hearing the commotion, the father ran into the room and managed to drag his enraged son away from his wife. He told us afterwards in the ward round that the attack had been ferocious. It was as if his son was possessed by some demonic strength. The mother said she believed her son at that time had wanted to kill her.

This takes place on the Wednesday afternoon ward round. The clinical team is attending, registrars or specialists in training, clinical psychologists, the social worker and the occupational therapist, the medical and nursing students and myself. The father and mother and daughter seem huddled together, as if these events have isolated them from a world that is no longer familiar or secure. The mother is crying. Rather absurdly, she apologises. The psychologist offers a tissue. The daughter watches her mother anxiously. The father appears stoical, or tries to be. For a while there is silence. I worry if this is the right way to help the family, a group of strangers bearing witness to their anguish. But they say they want to go on, they want us to understand what has happened so that maybe we can help.

I ask a rather odd question, but one that is often useful in trying to come to a meaningful diagnosis. 'It might be a strange thing to ask, but does it seem to you that in some way your son is a different person, that this is not Jannes?'

The mother becomes animated. 'Yes,' she says emphatically, 'yes, certainly. That's right. This is not my son. I want Jannes back. This is not who he is.'

The father and daughter nod in fierce agreement. So, this is not Jannes. But what has happened to him? Where is he, I wonder, when he eventually joins us and gazes upon me with disconcertingly vacant eyes.

Perhaps this is one of the greatest difficulties for the family: he is there and he is not there. He is young. He is healthy. There is no outward indication that he might be profoundly ill. There is no clear understanding about where this illness might be, where in his body or his mind.

The diagnosis – of mental illness, of psychosis or of schizophrenia

– is based on a characteristic cluster of clinical features, including delusions and hallucinations, various forms of thought disorders, social withdrawal, a restriction or blunting of emotions and a loss of volition. It represents a clinical syndrome rather than a diagnosis based on an objectively verifiable biological abnormality. This necessarily conventional description is insufficient, certainly beyond the confines of medicine, in the lived experience of those living with schizophrenia and their families. It gives little account of what is encountered as a calamity.

On another of the Wednesday-afternoon ward rounds, Dzunisani's wife is describing the events that led to his admission. She speaks in the present tense, in a soft voice, as if in a trance. 'He is on top of me … it is night … his hands are on my neck … I think I am going to die … I push him … away … I run for the door … I collect my children … I run from the house … the children are screaming … they are so afraid … he takes a knife … he comes after me … witch, he says, witch.' He was not himself, she tells us. He was a gentle man, a pastor in the local church. Now he is better. He is himself again. She doesn't know how he has achieved this recovery but she is grateful.

Dzunisani is appalled by what happened. He loves his wife. He doesn't want to kill her. That is inconceivable. She is not a witch. We ask him what he makes of it. He is unsure. 'It's the past. It's over. Perhaps it was some sort of devil possession. But I must go now. I must continue my pastoral work.' Perhaps to placate us, to persuade us that it is safe to discharge him, he promises to take the medication. I don't think any of us share his confidence. He does not know what caused this to happen. He does not consider it to be an illness, certainly not in a biological sense – why should he then take the medication? It is more probable that prayer would help him. It was just perhaps some sort of spiritual lapse. It seems likely that he will eventually stop the treatment. He will relapse, the symptoms will recur, and the lives of his wife and children will again be at risk. We tell the pastor and his wife of our concerns. She says she will do what she can.

But she is not sure. She cannot be. She is clearly troubled. What possible sense could be made of her husband not being himself, and now being himself again, and how could she ever again be sure?

It might be considered that there is some correspondence between schizophrenia and either personality disorders or dementias, but the schizophrenia spectrum disorders are fundamentally different. Personality and its disorders are variously described, but an intrinsic characteristic is a degree of continuity. Personalities, and personality disorders, do not change significantly after adolescence. X has a confident, cheerful disposition. Y tends to be moody and introspective. These patterns have a degree of predictability: X and Y are more likely than not to demonstrate these characteristics in a range of circumstances and at different times. This is in dramatic contrast to the stories of Jannes and Dzunisani. What their families described was a profoundly disturbing change of personality. This has nothing to do with a 'split' in personality. There are no different personalities or selves, but rather a loss of the integrity of the self.

Being no longer oneself is also described in the advanced stages of dementia. 'Dementia praecox' was used in the nineteenth and early twentieth centuries, prior to the adoption of the term 'schizophrenia' and then 'schizophrenia spectrum disorders'. But dementia and schizophrenia are again fundamentally different. Perhaps the most important distinguishing feature of the dementias is their relentlessly progressive nature. The initial indication might be forgetfulness, often considered a benign feature of aging. But as the dementia develops the deterioration is increasingly pervasive. First memory, then all cognitive functions, the capacity for feeling and being able to behave in an effective and socially responsible manner are cruelly eroded. Progression to death is the certain outcome. This is not schizophrenia, which is broadly conceived of as a neurodevelopmental disorder. The dementias are neurodegenerative disorders. The more characteristic course of the schizophrenia spectrum is a pattern of relapses and remissions.

It should not be assumed that delusions indicate schizophrenia, and certainly in the southern African context there needs to be great caution in ascribing a delusional process to beliefs that might be consistent with a person's cultural background. The delusions more consistent with a diagnosis of a delusional disorder tend to more plausible and of a less bizarre nature.

Angus insisted his wife was having an affair. She was a very conservative middle-aged woman and she found this as preposterous as it was distressing. He resorted to the most ludicrous, contorted arguments to justify his beliefs and became extremely agitated when challenged. He had threatened her with violence, and this had led to the admission. There were no features to suggest anything other than a delusional disorder. This encapsulated delusion was rigid and entrenched. We could not shift it but nevertheless she refused to consider a separation. She thought he was sick and that he needed her. He was her husband, she said. She did not say he was not the same man. She did not use the language of asking us to bring him back – but she was angry and sad and bewildered. Eventually a compromise was reached, but I was not confident that it could be sustained. He told us, and in a way we were impressed by his honesty, that he continued to believe in the affair but maybe this was something of the past and perhaps at some stage in the future he could consider forgiving her.

Gerhardus was not psychotic, but the stories he told us had no basis in his present reality. He had no short-term memory. The parts of his brain that subserved this vital function had been destroyed by alcohol. When I asked him what he had done over the weekend he had no idea. To fill the void he took recourse to memories of a more distant, happier, past. He was helpless, incapacitated by his amnesia, drifting through what remained of his life trapped in a bubble of the perpetual present. He was not deluded. The stories he made up of the past were not fixed in any way, but desperate strategies to orientate and retrieve himself. He was his old illusory self, living in the moment, enjoying too many beers with his mates, out on a boat somewhere, entirely content with his re-imagined circumstances.

There are no such consolations in schizophrenia. There are no such confabulations to grant a degree of respite. Too often there just seems to be an emptiness with nothing to fill it, a distraught mother pleading for her son's return.

34

I can't go on like this

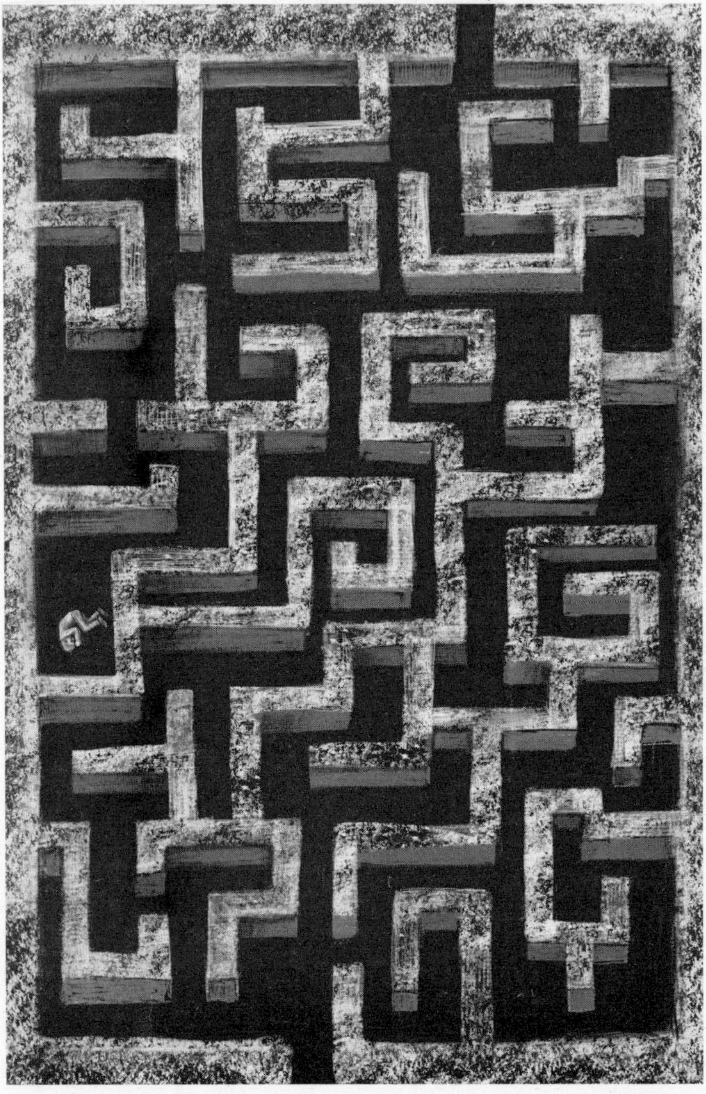

I can't go on like this. I have had it, Doctor. I don't know what to do now. Where is the end to it? I am on my own. There is nobody I can turn to. Everybody has given up trying to help. Maybe they blame me. They think it is my fault that he is like this. They think I must have done something wrong. His father has gone. He said it is either him or me. How can he expect me to make a choice like that? It is so cruel. It is so selfish. I need him but now he has left and he has got a new girlfriend and he wants nothing to do with us. He says the hospital must sort it out. He says the boy is sick and he is not a doctor or a nurse and it is not his responsibility. And now my daughter is suffering. She is afraid of her brother and she does not understand it is a sort of illness. She is being teased at school. She says the other children mock her and say that her brother is mad as if it is the whole family that is mad and they think his strange behaviour is funny because they don't have to live with it and they don't know how frightening it can be. She is a bright child but now she is failing the subjects she was good at. The teachers say she is not paying attention in class and they get angry with her. How can they understand what we are going through? Now she says she wants to change schools, but how will that help? It will be the same thing at another school. It is terrible that she is ashamed of her brother but I can understand it, I suppose. She is still too young to know that this is because of an illness but it is difficult anyway because he doesn't look ill. It's not as if he has a broken leg or is coughing with tuberculosis or dying of something. He is strong and healthy and so people don't believe he is sick so they don't feel any sympathy for him or for me. If it is not my fault, they say, it must be his. It is something he has done to himself. Maybe it is the drugs. Maybe he is being punished for something bad that he has done. When I say to them that the doctors have told me it is schizophrenia they say they don't know what that means as if they don't believe there is such a thing and it is perhaps just a word the doctors have invented to cover up bad behaviour or a mother not knowing how to discipline her child. In the beginning everybody was giving me advice but nothing helped. They said I should go and see a traditional healer. He said it was *amafufunyana* and that somebody had put a curse on him. I gave him the medicines and we had to do some things but it didn't work. He got worse so I took him back to the healer and then he said perhaps it was *ukuthwasa*, that he was being called to be a healer, but I don't know about those things and then anyway my boy said he would not go back to the healer and nothing came of it. Nothing was helping and I was becoming desperate. Then people said I must just throw him out but how can I do that? He is a child. He is sick. He would not survive. There is nobody else now except me and I don't know how to cope any longer. I know you doctors are trying to help and I know you can't just keep him in hospital forever but what am I supposed to do? It's so sad. He is quite well when he comes out of the hospital but it does not last for very long. He has no friends. Nobody wants to see him. They just see him now as a mad person and they are embarrassed when he tries to approach them. They laugh at him and run away. It is understandable that he gets angry. It is not his fault, he says, this illness. He did not ask for it. It is too unfair. Then he starts with the drugs because he is angry and lonely so then the only people who will have anything to do with him are the gangsters. They use his disability grant to get the drugs and they don't care if the drugs make him sick so that he has to go back to hospital. I am so afraid. He is going to get into trouble because of these gangsters and then he is going to end up in prison and then there will really be no hope. I am afraid of these people. They come into the house and they show no respect for me. They know that I am on my own and they will start stealing from me for the drugs and the police will do nothing because they say they have more important things to deal with and anyway it is my son's fault because he invites them into the house. Things are just getting worse and worse and Doctor it is terrible to say this but sometimes I just wish he was dead. How can a mother say that about her son? It is wrong. I will be punished but it is the truth. Either him or me. I would rather be dead than go on like this. Last night it was just too much. I knew it was going to happen at some point. I knew it was coming. So I locked the door and my daughter was with me. How can one live like that, in fear of your own son? But this time I was really afraid. He had been behaving strangely all afternoon and I couldn't reach him. He was so angry. He was in a rage but he would not tell me or he couldn't tell me what the matter was. Perhaps it was the drugs. We, my daughter and myself, locked ourselves in the bedroom but we couldn't really sleep and in the early hours of the morning he started hammering at the door and screaming things that I did not understand. My daughter started screaming also, she was so afraid. He went on and on. He wouldn't stop even though I was pleading with him through the door to leave us alone. Then he started to kick at the door. It is not a strong door and I knew he was going to break it down. He came into the room and he was ranting at me and he was carrying a knife from the kitchen in his hand. He was mad. He shouted at me 'You witch!' There was hatred in his eyes and I thought he was going to kill me. I just screamed his name and said, 'Leave us, please leave us!' Then he just stood there as if in a daze. My daughter was sobbing in terror. A neighbour must have been woken by all this noise and started hammering at the front door and shouted that the police had been called. My son just stood there shaking, and when the police did come he went with them without complaining or fighting with them. He seemed like a little boy then, obedient, no longer the mad dangerous person he had just been. So now he is in hospital and we feel safe for a little while and we can sleep at last but I know you are going to discharge him when he is well enough and this is all going to start again. I don't know what to do any longer, Doctor. I can't go on like this.

I can't go on like this. Last night was the worst. It was terrible. I was frightened. I don't know what was going on. I think I nearly killed my mother. How could that have happened. I was out of control. Everything was muddled. I didn't think she was my mother. I thought she was somebody that was pretending to be my mother. I thought she was an imposter and I was angry and frightened. I thought she was a witch. This suddenly became clear to me. I knew it. I knew that she was why everything was going wrong in my life. I felt I had to do this thing, that I did not have any choice. I took the knife from the kitchen and I went to her bedroom. She had locked the door and this made me even more angry. I was in some sort of uncontrollable rage. It was almost as if some force had taken control over me and was driving me to do these things. I was not myself. Maybe I was possessed. I smashed down the door. I saw that my mother was terrified. So was my little sister. My mother shouted my name. She shouted, 'Leave us, please leave us!' I became confused. Perhaps it was her calling my name and seeing my sister being so afraid. I felt horrible. I did not know what was going on again. I was not sure whether this woman who might have been my mother was a witch or not. Nothing was clear or certain. Then maybe I thought something had happened to me, that I had become sick again and that I needed help. In a way it was a relief that the police came. It was too dangerous. I could have killed my mother. How would I have been able to live with that? How can I live with that? I don't understand this illness. The doctors call it schizophrenia but what does that mean? It is not a sickness that I can understand. It is not that I have got an infection or a broken leg or anything like that that the doctors can fix. They say that it is a problem with my brain but I don't get fits. I don't get headaches. I feel well. I am healthy. What kind of sickness is this? There were no problems when I was younger. Things were just fine. I am not sure when or how it started. I think it was a problem at school. There never had been a problem but I started to have difficulties in concentrating and I started struggling and the teachers got angry with me. They said I was being lazy. Then my friends started teasing me. They said I was weird. I didn't know what they were talking about but I became unsure of myself and things got worse and then I had no friends and people were laughing at me and calling me mad. I stopped going to school. My father got angry. He said, 'What is the matter with you?' but I didn't know and he hit me. My mother tried to stop him and then he left. He said we were all mad and he had to look after himself. I felt so ashamed. My mother took me to all sorts of people who said all sorts of weird things. They said somebody had put a curse on me. Then they said I was being called to become a healer. I don't believe all that stuff but I didn't know what was going on and then I wasn't sure of anything. My mother took me to the local clinic and the doctor there said she thought it was maybe this thing called schizophrenia and referred us to a specialist doctor at the hospital. I refused to go. I didn't want to be called a mad person. I was not mad. I didn't want to be sick. I didn't want this to be happening. But I couldn't stop it. I began to notice strange things. It was odd and it made me anxious. It was as if I was getting signals but I did not know where they came from or what these signals meant. Things became blurred, they were no longer what they seemed to be. I could not understand it and then I began to think that people were playing tricks on me. Why should people be doing this to me? I had not hurt anybody. Why? It was so unfair. This got worse. I became afraid. I did not want to leave the house. Then one night I just lost control completely. I don't know what happened. Maybe I was possessed by the devil. I was just screaming and bashing my head against the wall so that there was blood everywhere. Maybe I was trying to kill something inside me. I don't know but it was bad and I was terrified. I ended up in hospital and that was also frightening. I thought the other people there were mad. They gave me some medicines and things got better and I was sent home. I didn't like taking the medication. I felt better and I didn't think I needed that stuff. Why should you take medicines if you are not sick? It made me think that maybe I was sick in some strange way that I didn't know and that made it worse. I did not believe that I would be sick again if I stopped the treatment. I refused to believe it. I am a young person. My life is ahead of me. I don't want to be sick. I am not mad. Maybe it was just the stress of the problems at school and my friends but

I am over that now, I think. The social worker made an application for a disability grant because they said I had a mental illness and would not be able to work. That made me depressed but my mother said it would help because there was very little money and no support from my father. I had no friends but the gangsters started coming around to the house. At first I thought they were quite cool. They made me think that I belonged but I suppose it was just the money from the grant that they wanted. They gave me drugs and that was also quite cool. It made me feel strong. It made me think I could do anything and that I wasn't sick in any way and that I didn't need the medicines. Then it all started going wrong again and it was worse and this terrible thing happened and now I am back in the hospital. I feel bad. I feel very guilty. I look at my mother and I see how disappointed she is and how tired and angry she is and I don't know what I can do to help her and my little sister. I feel like such a failure. Sometimes I think I would rather be dead. I don't know how I can go on like this.

35

Odd ideas, and rarely a strange beauty

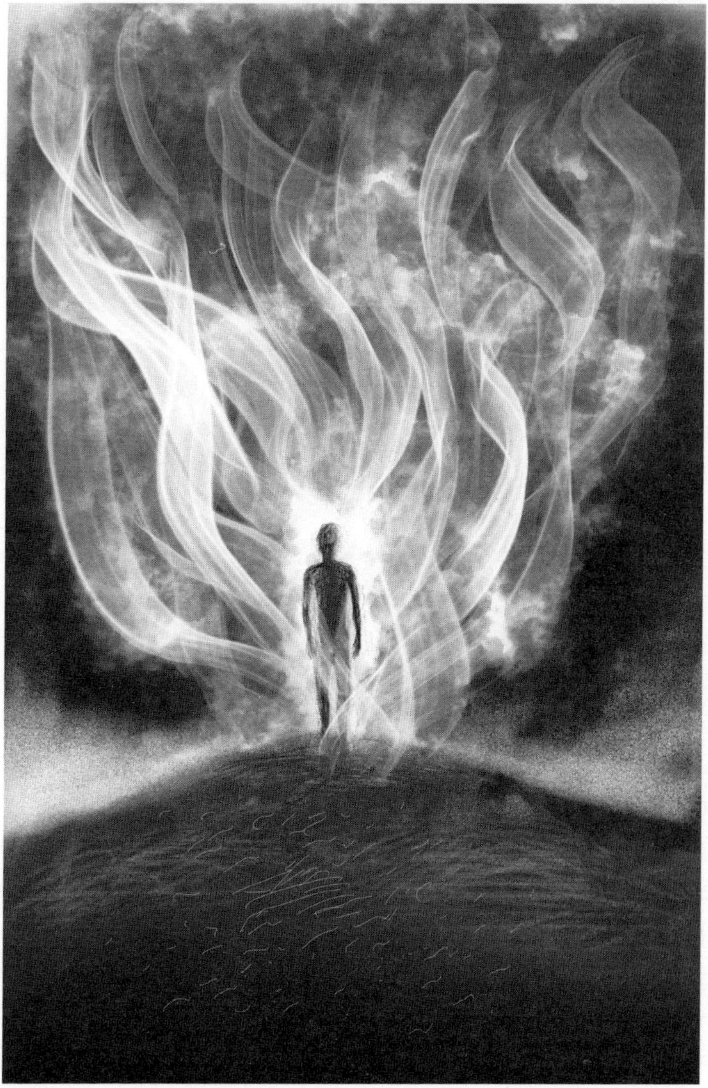

Reuben greets me affably. He could have been considered handsome but he clearly pays no heed to his appearance. He shakes my hand but the left hand is stuck down the front of his dirty trousers. After a few polite and formal exchanges, I ask him why he is doing this. He laughs and says he is fine and there is nothing that I should worry about. I persist. He insists that there is no problem. I say that it is odd to put your hand down the front of your trousers, it is inappropriate. I hesitate but do not say that others will think he is crazy. He laughs again, and says, as if taking me into his confidence, 'You see, I have to. I must hold onto my penis all the time.'

'Why?' And this time I say, 'People will think you have got a problem and turn away from you. You might scare them. What's going on?'

Laughter again. 'You must understand, I have to hold on because my mother has her hand rammed up my rectum. She is trying to rip off my penis.' Then, as if to reassure me, he repeats: 'It's okay. I'm all right. As long as I hold on tight she can't do it. I'm fine, really.' And then, quite kindly: 'Don't worry, Doc. There's nothing wrong with me. I can cope.'

I ask for his permission to speak to his mother. She is a charming, immaculately dressed woman in her middle age. She is exhausted. She says this is a relatively good phase, because he is calm and he is polite to her. When things get bad, she says, he rages against her. He accuses her of trying to castrate him. His language is obscene and vituperative. He is violent. She fears for her life. She is resigned, she tells me. She thinks that probably one day he will kill her.

Matricide is a rare event, and when it does occur it is most often in this context. It is as if these young men living with schizophrenia find themselves in an intolerable trap. They cannot live without the mother and the mother is perceived as suffocating them, stifling them, castrating them, not allowing them to live and be free. The only – albeit psychotic – solution to this problem is to kill the mother or kill themselves. In this there is no strange beauty, only a relentless, enervating horror. She has lost her son but he is there, tormenting her, threatening her, and when she has gone who will look after him? Who other than a mother could bear this burden?

The mothers seem to most often bear the brunt of this. The fathers tend to withdraw or to flee, as do the siblings. Jan, in a quite similar way, was violent towards his mother. He is an exceptionally bright young man, but in late adolescence he became withdrawn. His academic performance declined and eventually to his parents' great distress he refused to go to school. The situation deteriorated steadily until it became clear that he was gravely ill. He assaulted his mother, accusing her of having sex with the gardener. Then in a rage he accused her of trying to have sex with him. She was aghast. The family struggled on until it seemed that something had to give. The father said, 'I can't go on like this. It is either him or me.' The mother felt she had no choice. The father left, and so did the younger brother. When she brought Jan to see me, she was trying to cope on her own.

Jan was unlike Reuben. He was distracted, perplexed and angry. He lacked the possibly protective nature of Reuben's apparent calm. There is no stereotype of schizophrenia, but Reuben did show some of its curiously characteristic features. He described what must have been an excruciating experience in the form of a somatic or bodily and persecutory delusion. The corresponding manifest emotion or affect was nevertheless, for the most part, a curiously bland indifference. Another feature he demonstrated was an extremely concrete way of thinking and acting. He was incapable of understanding that the experiences he described could have no basis in reality. That this could be construed as a delusion was beyond his capacity for abstraction. Furthermore, there was a simple, concrete solution to the problem. He just had to hold onto his penis. Then everything, for the time being, would be all right.

This failure of an abstracting ability might itself seem an unhelpful abstraction in the attempt to make sense of the array of symptoms associated with the schizophrenia spectrum, and the corresponding havoc that ensues in the decline in functioning. A loss of the capacity for abstraction is part of a cluster of cognitive deficits loosely described as impairments of executive functioning. This is variously defined, but includes – in addition to the problems of abstraction – a difficulty in formulating goals and planning accordingly, of sequencing, problem-solving and evaluating. It is difficult to comprehend the devastating impact this has on young people's lives. Both Reuben and Jan had become helpless. Unable to plan, to consider the future, to reflect and adapt, they were at sea, at the mercy of circumstances they perceived to be either entirely out of their control or cruelly menacing.

The term 'executive function' does little to convey the dramatic impact of its impairments. The capacity to function in a way that is dependent on intact executive functioning is at the core of what it might be to be considered personhood, to be able to act intentionally, to be self-reflective, to imagine.

This absence or loss of executive function is in stark contrast to the delusions and hallucinations that are more characteristic of the 'positive' features of schizophrenia. Positive and negative forms have different pathophysiological bases and tend to have different prognoses. The difference is such that the notion of schizophrenia as a clinical entity is questionable, and the term 'schizophrenia spectrum disorder' is considered more appropriate. Positive and negative forms are furthermore not discrete, and may commingle.

I asked Xanta what he did during the day. He said, quite placidly, 'Nothing.' I said he must surely do something, maybe wander about, occasionally prepare a meal, sleep and wake up. 'No,' he said, not emphatically, but blandly, unperturbed, 'nothing, I do nothing.'

'But surely you do not spend the entire day just staring at the wall?'

'Yes, that's what I do. I stare at the wall.'

'Don't you get bored?'

He thought for a moment. Perhaps he sensed that in some way he had disappointed me and that I needed reassurance.

'Sometimes I get frightened.'

Just a fear, no sense of even the slightest pleasure, no other emotion filled his empty days.

This strange flatness of emotion, this perplexing lack of responsiveness, an absence of being present can understandably be the most distressing aspect of the illness to family members. It can also not be interpreted as part of an illness, and this tends to happen in deprived households where overcrowding and a multitude of stresses result in the solitary, vacant young man in the corner simply being neglected, for weeks and for months, until some dramatic event – a TV being destroyed, for example – leads to a panicked call for help. This smashing of TVs is a curiously common occurrence and, for Xanta, arises from the belief that characters in a drama are addressing him directly and abusively. It represents an eruption of positive symptoms in the form of delusions from the otherwise empty and featureless terrain of schizophrenia.

Hasim's response to his vivid delusions was less impassive than bemused. When I saw him in the outpatient clinic he told me that things had improved considerably. He was smiling, almost to himself – as if, with some distance that had developed between himself and his illness, he found the whole process quite fascinating. The briars patch, he told me, was slowly fading into background radiation. I asked him what the briars patch might be. He said it was a zone in his bedroom inhabited by a creature resembling a giant octopus. 'When I'm schizophrenic this malevolent creature shoots out tentacles. These things jam into my mouth so that I cannot breathe.' He laughed. 'It's mad,' he said. 'It's terrible. It's just not cricket.'

Laughter helps, sometimes. Nicholas told us that his goal in life was to set up an ice-hockey team in Australia. We told him we thought that was a crazy idea because Australia was a very hot country. He said that was not a problem. He would simply cast a spell on it to make it cold. He laughed. It was such a simple solution. Could we not understand? We asked him whether he could not rather cast a spell for rain, as the province was experiencing a severe drought at the time. He laughed again. That was not at all a concern for him. The ice rink in Australia was the big issue.

But more often, there is no laughter. While the disjunction between the content of thinking and the associated emotional tone is suggestive of the diagnosis of schizophrenia, it is the ensuing behaviour that most often raises the alarm and leads to a hospital admission. For Nxaba, who had tried to burn down his family's shack and was plagued by gangsters for his disability grant, the situation was dangerous. His mother wondered whether her son had tried to burn down the shack so that there would be nothing left for the gangsters to take. Was this his sort of solution?

In such circumstances, it seems that the alternative, more unperturbed, responses to psychotic phenomena are preferable and provide at least a degree of protection. Adriaan is pleasant but vague in his manner towards us. He is not distressed at all by the issues that have led to his admission. It is not a problem that his twin brother is not even his brother, let alone his twin. He is 'quite nice', this other person. He seems to be quite caring. His mother is not his mother, but whoever she is she is also 'quite nice'. Although he does not seem to think that this is a problem, his mother certainly does.

During the interview with Adriaan, I assume a posture of confusion. 'I don't understand. I can't understand how you can refuse to accept that this woman who brought you into the world and who has cared for you all your life is your mother.'

The disavowal is rigid. He gazes at me placidly, and asks, as if it is a matter of some debate, 'Do you believe in parents?'

I respond, 'Surely it is not a matter of belief. It is a biological fact of life. Children are born of parents.'

He is utterly unimpressed. It is simply a matter of belief, as is everything. He is imbued with a strange contentment, or maybe an indifference, as if all the world and everything that happens is not a given but chosen, to be believed or not believed. This is possibly his way of regaining control. His impassivity makes him impervious to hurt, as it does to the disappointment and dismay surrounding him.

That there should be any sort of strange beauty in these accounts might seem improbable, if not preposterous. Any attempt to romanticise serious mental illness should be fiercely guarded against, and is more likely to do harm than good. It is ignorant and fails to register the gravity and the great distress of those living with schizophrenia and their families and communities. Yet while acknowledging this I find it difficult not to see, in these struggles to make sense of a confounding and often terrifying world, a strange grace and an unexpected beauty. These stories do, in a way, represent determined, often convoluted and bizarre but inventive strategies to survive, and to find some sort of solution, albeit psychotic, to the otherwise overwhelming problem of noise and meaninglessness.

36

Hearing voices, or listening

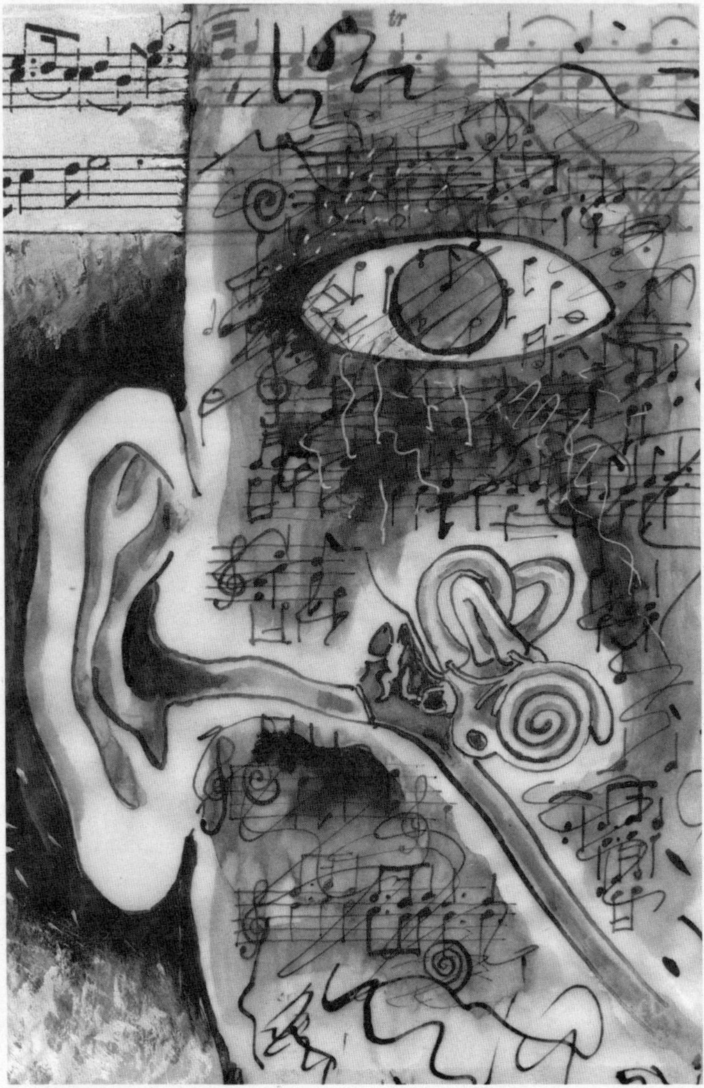

'When I'm sick the machine comes on … the voices are clearer … there is no barrier … I was too much into this thing to question it … it would drive me completely insane … it's a man's worst nightmare … this remote brain control … there's no escaping it. It is complex … how can I describe it … it's like snowing on TV … it's a sensation like that … it's the closest I can describe … it's not just what you visualise.' – Tsebo, describing a psychotic episode from which he has recently recovered

Hearing voices, or having auditory hallucinations, is considered to be a core feature of psychosis – of schizophrenia more specifically. Hearing voices does not indicate madness. We all, in certain circumstances, have the capacity to hear voices or noises that have no correspondence to the external world. This needs to be emphasised, as a misinterpretation of hallucinations has too often led to false diagnoses with baleful consequences. Voices or noises are perceived to arise in external space. The voice of God or the ancestors, or the voice of reason or conscience experienced internally, are of course not hallucinations and thus not evidence of madness.

A further distinction that is not sufficiently emphasised in the academic literature is the distress associated with these phenomena. Tsebo describes his experience as the 'worst nightmare'. Hearing voices should not necessarily be distressing. The patient who informed us that the voices he heard were enquiring whether they could befriend him on Facebook described being quite content. The voices were companionable, and he saw no reason why they should be extinguished and nor did we.

Clearly it is inadequate to consider that hearing voices is in itself inherently pathological. For Tsebo the anguish seemed to arise more specifically from the belief that he was no longer in control. There was no barrier between himself and the outside world. He had become engulfed by these external stimuli which because they were beyond his control were understandably all the more intolerable.

Samuel regarded himself as being most fortunate to be alive, and so did we. He had been found by his mother after trying to hang himself from a clothing hook behind a bedroom door. She had heard a crashing sound, presumably due to the weight of his body having dislodged the hook, and found him collapsed and blue in the face but alive. He had been behaving strangely for some days or weeks. He had become withdrawn and his appearance was ill-kempt. His mother had attributed this to adolescent problems. This occurs frequently – it is a turbulent period. Perhaps he had been bullied at school, perhaps he had been rebuffed by a girlfriend, but whatever the reason what is familiar to any parent is the child's reluctance to divulge what might have caused the change in behaviour.

Samuel was remarkably frank with us in the immediate aftermath of his attempted suicide. He said he did not want to die. He had had no intention of killing himself. He had everything to live for. The problem was the voices. This had started some weeks earlier, and initially was almost imperceptible, more an unfamiliar noise than any signal that he might be becoming ill. The voices had become gradually more intense, crystallising into discernible words that then became derogatory and abusive. As he slowly crashed into psychosis he described the voices as incessant and increasingly commanding. He was told that he was worthless and deserved to die. He struggled to resist but the voices became too powerful. His will, his fundamental instinct for survival, was eroded. As for Tsebo, it seemed to him then that he had no option but to end his life. Sitting up in his hospital bed, fully recovered, in recounting these events he seemed bemused, as if this could not possibly have happened to him – that in some mystifying way it must have been somebody else.

Describing these phenomena as auditory hallucinations seems inadequate. The aridly objective, notionally academic term gives no indication of the distress associated with the voices or the behavioural consequences. The associated phenomena are closer to the core of what a patient might be experiencing and closer to what might be considered to be the priorities in terms of a therapeutic intervention. It was not the voices in themselves that prompted such anguish with disastrous consequences, but the disruption of something beyond, and something that might be considered innate and particularly human: a sense of self, of the privacy of the self, and a precarious notion of free will.

This chapter is ostensibly about hearing voices, but the argument is that it is not possible – and that it is a distortion – to separate voices from the other, intimately associated, psychotic phenomena that afflict our patients. A person does not complain of hearing voices in isolation. If this might happen on the rare occasion, it is unlikely that it would indicate the need for any form of intervention.

Tsebo described being 'too much into this thing to question it'. This shows insight into a loss of insight. The term 'psychosis' is variously defined. It might be described as being characterised by delusions and hallucinations and thought disorders, or a common denominating feature might be articulated as a loss of insight. This is in itself problematic. Insight is a matter of degree, not an absolute, and requires qualification. For example, in presenting a patient to the consultant a registrar might say, 'He shows some insight into the idea that he might be ill but has no insight into the need for treatment.' On whose authority insight or a lack thereof might be defined may be open to dispute. It might also be presumptuous to consider an absence of insight as being limited to the mentally ill – as if those of us unburdened with such labels have a clear and unremitting insight into the vagaries of our thinking and behaviour, or are incapable of self-deception. Coupled to a lack of insight, a defining characteristic of psychosis is that beliefs are held with conviction despite evidence to the contrary. Clinicians are wearisomely familiar with the indignant complaint, 'What am I doing here? There is nothing wrong with me.'

Tsebo described being bombarded with electric shocks from outer space. These bolts were intensely painful and were all the more distressing because he could not understand where they came from and why he was being persecuted in this way. He became increasingly agitated while telling me this. 'I know what you are thinking, Doctor,' he said. 'I know you think this is delusional, I know you think this is a relapse of the schizophrenia. But it's not. It's real. It's happening to me, and it's terrible.' He was, as he said in retrospect, 'too much into it', too overwhelmed by it to question whether it might be an expression of his illness. At the time, however, he did show a degree of insight, being acutely aware of what I was thinking, prompting his indignant and pained response.

Again, in this respect the term 'insight' seems insufficient and requires elaboration to gain some idea of what a person might be experiencing. In these accounts patients have described being trapped. What they describe is not a hypothesis – it represents a brutal reality. There are no other ways of seeing it, no metaphorical spaces.

The source or the cause of these disturbing phenomena remains elusive. Functional scanning indicates that the hallucinations are self-generated. What a person is saying, without sound, appears to be perceived in external space. Voices are most often in the third person, commenting on a person's thoughts or actions. 'Look at what he is doing now: he has these bad thoughts now, he is bad.' Quite often ceaseless and maddeningly intrusive, they extend to commands: 'He is so bad that he really should not be alive,' and then, 'Go on, do it.'

Tsebo described the experience as 'snowing' on a television screen. This seems an apt metaphor for an auditory perception. Snow is the visual equivalent of noise. There is no signal, no meaningful pattern. The world makes no sense. There is no integrity, no continuity, no coherence, no means of making sense. It is the 'worst nightmare'.

If the notion of a psychosis is un-understandable by definition, what might be more understandable is the quite desperate struggle to make sense of the experience of noise, to mitigate it, to create a familiar pattern that might restore a sense of control and a degree of equanimity. It is also understandable that these strategies might derive from one's social or cultural context. This is why in the middle-class suburbs of the city a frequent complaint was that characters on television were talking to one personally, and why young men from rural backgrounds often described the voices as being those of displeased ancestors.

The biological basis for this perception of noise is uncertain. The neural correlates indicated by brain imaging might provide some indication. There is neural activity, but a loss of signal. Music might be a useful metaphor. What is perceived as synchronous or beautiful or joyful is the expression of an extremely complex orchestrated process. A symphony, for example, consists of a wide range of instruments being played with great skill to a score and under the supervising coordination of a conductor. In the audience we do not attend to the component parts, except perhaps when things go wrong. We celebrate the totality of it. We imagine we grasp the intent of the composer, enabled by the skill of the players and the conductor. All is harmonious. In the context of auditory perception all makes sense. But as this is a highly complex, intricate process, things can go wrong. The first violinist has omitted to take his medication for an attention deficit hyperactivity disorder. He rushes ahead, ignoring the desperate attempts of the conductor to restrain him. The oboe player has fallen asleep. The percussionist, eager to impress the pretty second violinist, overreaches himself on the kettle drum. The delicate balance is lost. The music becomes noise.

Clearly, in a biological context there are levels of explanation. A current plausible model for psychosis is a dysconnectivity syndrome, or a dysregulation of the elaborate and dynamic web of synaptic connections in the central nervous system – a disorganisation of the orchestra. The underlying causes of this dysregulation are indeterminate, but probably concern the shifting and complex interactions of genetic and environmental factors. This is not discontinuous with what occurs in a healthy brain in the process of perception. On the basis of very limited sensory information and past experience, we make inferences about what we might consider to be the most likely percept. The voice I hear and that speaks to me in a coherent and meaningful way is not a vibration of air molecules or the agitation of hair cells in the inner ear. The voice and the meaning I attach to its utterances are internally represented or constructed. It seems that this inferential process is what goes awry in psychotic states.

The way in which hallucinations – and more generally psychoses – are conceptualised has important implications for how they are managed. Within a strictly reductive biomedical model the hallucinations are symptoms of a pathological process. The content of the voices, and the person's experience and his or her response to these voices, are not relevant. The implication is that an appropriate treatment goal should be the elimination of the troublesome symptom. What the person might make of this is not clear and is not taken into account. 'It's just a symptom of the schizophrenia. It will go away with treatment.' It is meaningless.

Alternatively, the symptom may be understood as the patient's attempt to make sense of his or her experience. This might be cautious and idiosyncratic, but in all likelihood represents a striving for an explanation that is personally and culturally meaningful – and if so this needs to be acknowledged, not necessarily suppressed. The decision to intervene requires careful consideration and should not merely be assumed. In this respect treatment in the form of the elimination of symptoms by pharmacological means may be experienced as a denial of one's tentative reality and an interruption of a potentially therapeutic process. The symptom is considered anomalous and invalid. This disregard could be a factor in the widely prevalent non-adherence to treatment.

For the young man from a rural background hearing voices might become listening to the ancestors. A pathological event is reconstrued as a culturally meaningful experience. It is validated. The young man is not ostracised. He is attuned; he is listening to the ancestors. This is contingent upon a particular set of cultural beliefs, of course, but the implication in general is that it might be more helpful and useful to our patients for us to listen to what they are telling us, rather than simply to suppress the symptoms of psychosis.

This is not an argument against pharmacological treatment, but an attempt to redefine the principles and goals of treatment. A focus of attention beyond signs and symptoms, and an endeavour to attend to the experience and concerns of a person living with schizophrenia, seems likely to be more acceptable, to be less likely to do harm, and to be more probably beneficial.

There is a world of difference between hearing and listening.

37

A family aghast

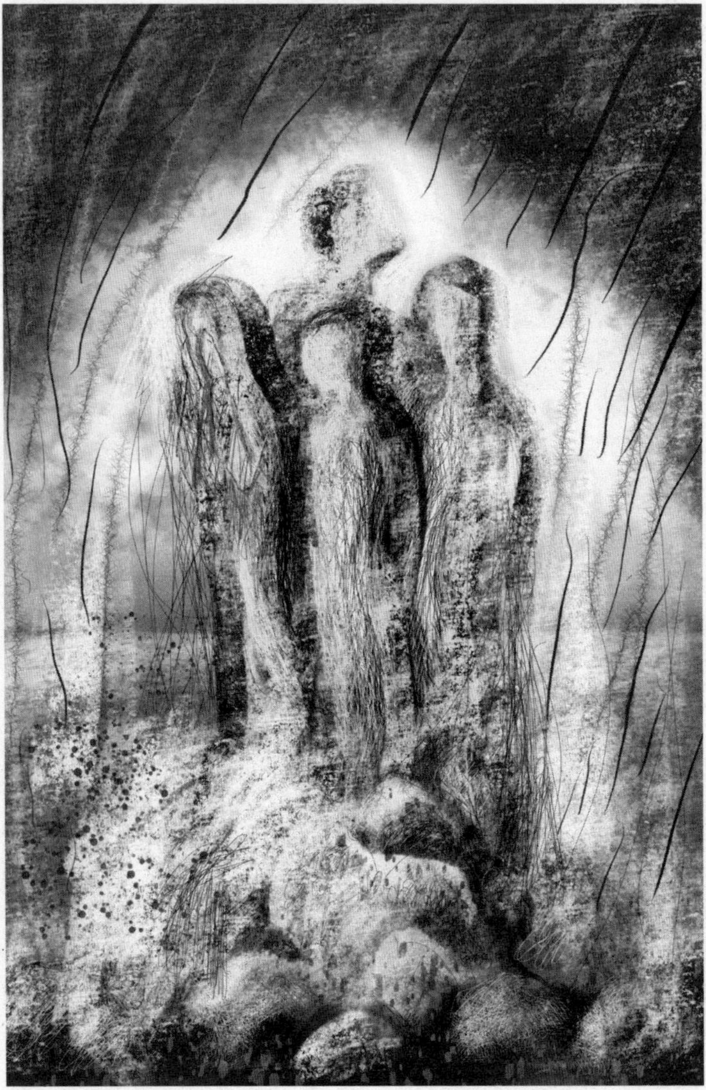

I have been fired by a patient. He is angry and arrogant. He swaggers about the admission ward. He is a big shot. He runs the show. His name is Sayid. He fires all and sundry, including his fellow patients. He bellows: 'You have to go. You are not up to it. I have to sort this mess out myself. All of you! Out! Now!' The staff are amused. The patients are bewildered. Who is this man? Why is he shouting at them? He is a patient. Who does he think he is?

This is what usually happens when Sayid comes in. The bravado does not last long. Things break down fairly quickly and then Sayid becomes tearful and anxious and abject. It is poignant. The puffed-up psychotic persona is perhaps something he imagines he should be, but it is unsustainable. He cannot be who he thinks he should be or who he thinks his mother and his extended family wish him to be.

We have known each other for a long time. He is a pleasant, intelligent young man who lives with an older brother and his parents in a quite affluent suburb of the city. He has lived with schizophrenia since his middle teenage years. He has coped relatively well and has only required two or three admissions to hospital. He attends the outpatient clinic and usually manages to be fairly cheerful and optimistic. His manner towards me is for the most part friendly and respectful. On these occasions it is unthinkable that, in an altered state, he might choose to fire me.

Probably in part because of his illness he did not achieve a matric pass. This does not seem to have deterred him unduly. He works for his father's building company and earns a small salary. He is clearly respected by his co-workers and he is loved by his family and admired for the way he has not allowed himself to become downcast by his illness. They are a conservative and devout Muslim family. They have undertaken to inform themselves as fully as possible about this strange illness and they are supportive of Sayid, encouraging him to take his medication and to attend the outpatient clinics and to be hopeful. They maintain understandably the expectation that maybe one day this might all pass and he will marry and have children and perhaps take over his father's business.

Sayid has a close relationship with his older brother, Mohammed. Generously, he has not allowed Mohammed's success to come between them. Mohammed did well at school, matriculated with a first-class pass and started a degree course in engineering at the university. He was the pride of his family and of the community. Sayid shared in this pride and showed no sign of resentment with regard to the greater attention inevitably shown to his elder brother.

It was in the second year of his degree that Mohammed began to show the first signs of illness. He became withdrawn, he isolated himself from his friends and his academic performance began to suffer. The course convener expressed concern. The family were appalled. This could not be happening, not again, not to their pride and joy. They hesitated. Things got worse. Mohammed stopped attending classes. He locked himself in his room. He started shouting in the night as if, it seemed to his horrified family, he was being terrorised by assailants. The situation became intolerable.

I am not sure why the decision was made to seek help in the private sector. Maybe the family believed the treatment would be superior to that of the public sector. Maybe there was some wishful thought that if he was treated in a different system there would be a different outcome.

He was seen in private by one of my colleagues who is also of the Muslim faith. The referral was not discussed with me so I do not know what transpired, but it seems possible that the family hoped that this psychiatrist would form an opinion that was different from my evaluation of his brother. It was not to be. A provisional diagnosis was made of schizophrenia. Medication was started. There was some degree of improvement and Mohammed returned with some hesitation to his classes.

Yet things could not be the same again. Everybody involved had become vigilant, anxious. What would happen? Would he be able to cope with the academic demands of his engineering course? Would it all be all right in the end? Would he follow the course of his younger brother? The family had coped with that as best they could, but also could not regard these events as anything but a sad and profound disappointment. How could they cope with having to go through this all over again with their only other child, their hope for the future? Please let this not be happening. Please would it go away.

A tense and fraught time ensued. Mohammed did not seem to be quite himself. There was a distracted way about him. The family attributed this to the traumatic events of the recent past and chose to believe that it would take time to recover. Patience and their love and support and their prayers would bring him through this ordeal.

I do not know what prompted the family at that point to embark on a pilgrimage. I do know that it is required by the faith, and that neither Sayid nor Mohammed had been on haj. I do not know whether the family hoped that the holy rituals of the pilgrimage might accelerate their troubled son's recovery. The family did not consult me, but there was no reason for me not to encourage the pilgrimage and when I saw Sayid before his departure he was full of excitement and anticipation.

The subsequent events are not clear and were reported to me by Sayid some time later when he was still in a highly emotional and distraught state. Initially the pilgrimage had been thrilling. The family had felt swept along by the enormous crowds and the clamour and an overwhelming sense of a collective religious fervour. I am not sure if this was all too much for Mohammed. I am not sure if, in an exulted religious state, he chose or merely omitted to take his medication. He became agitated and the family became anxious. The situation deteriorated rapidly. His increasingly disorganised behaviour could not in any way be interpreted as a state of spiritual transportation. Increasingly fearful for his safety, the family locked him in the hotel bedroom on the fifth floor of their luxury hotel. Left briefly unattended, Mohammed found an open window in the bathroom and threw himself to his death.

The family were aghast. Not only had they lost their beloved son in the holiest of places, but many of the faith believe strongly that suicide is sinful. There was to be no consolation that their son was on his way to heaven.

I could not address these issues with Sayid and his mother when I next saw them in the outpatient clinic. It did not seem appropriate and it was certainly not for me question an article of a faith that had sustained the family throughout their lives. On this occasion Sayid appeared to be putting on a brave front. He seemed to be determined to take on the role of his deceased elder brother. His manner was almost nonchalant. He showed no signs of grief. His mother just stared ahead. She scarcely spoke. The father did not attend. The mother said his spirit was broken.

Six months later the father was murdered. It appeared to be one of those random, brutal calamities that occur in the city. There had been an attempted robbery. The father had intervened to protect his property and in the ensuing struggle he had been stabbed to death.

In the conservative tradition of this bereft family, Sayid is now the head of the household. When I next see him his manner is even more inappropriate than when I saw him following his brother's suicide. He is determined to show that he is strong, that he can cope. He is bluff. He is blandly aloof. His manner towards his grieving mother is cruelly abrupt. He appears to be impatient with her and oblivious to the tears running down her cheeks. He wants to show that he is the head of the family, that he is in charge. It is sad and it is doomed. The mother, exhausted, shakes her head, nods, gestures as if to say it is all too predictable: he can't cope, of course; he is becoming sick and she does not know what to do.

The next time I see Sayid he has been admitted to our unit. He is indignant and enraged. He fires me and everybody else. Now he is on his own. There is no elder brother. There is no father. He stalks about the ward, slowly becoming uneasy, fearful of his vulnerability.

It will be like this, time and time again. He will recover and he will make a great effort to cope. He tries to make a success of his father's business but he does not have the skills or the resources. The business fails.

The mother and son have to leave the family home. It is too much. Things break down yet again and he is back with us, the king of the castle, the master of his tragic universe.

It seems possible that the psychosis is some sort of escape. He could fire me, perhaps loathing the role I play in his life. He could, for a while, imagine that things are not as they are, and that he is magnificently in control. I cannot remember him formally reappointing me, but after a few days he calms down and even shows a degree of contrition. There is no more swagger, no more bravado. He is then just a very troubled and anxious young man in a painfully difficult situation.

Eventually and reluctantly, on each of these occasions he accepts treatment. He gets better and he is discharged. Time passes; the mother comes back. She does not have to explain very much. 'It is all starting again. I can't manage.' I cannot say it will be all right. I ask her to sign the forms for an involuntary admission. We go through the cycle again. There can be no enduring alleviation of the predicament of this most unfortunate family. To presume otherwise is unhelpful and wrong.

38

Suicide and its aftermath

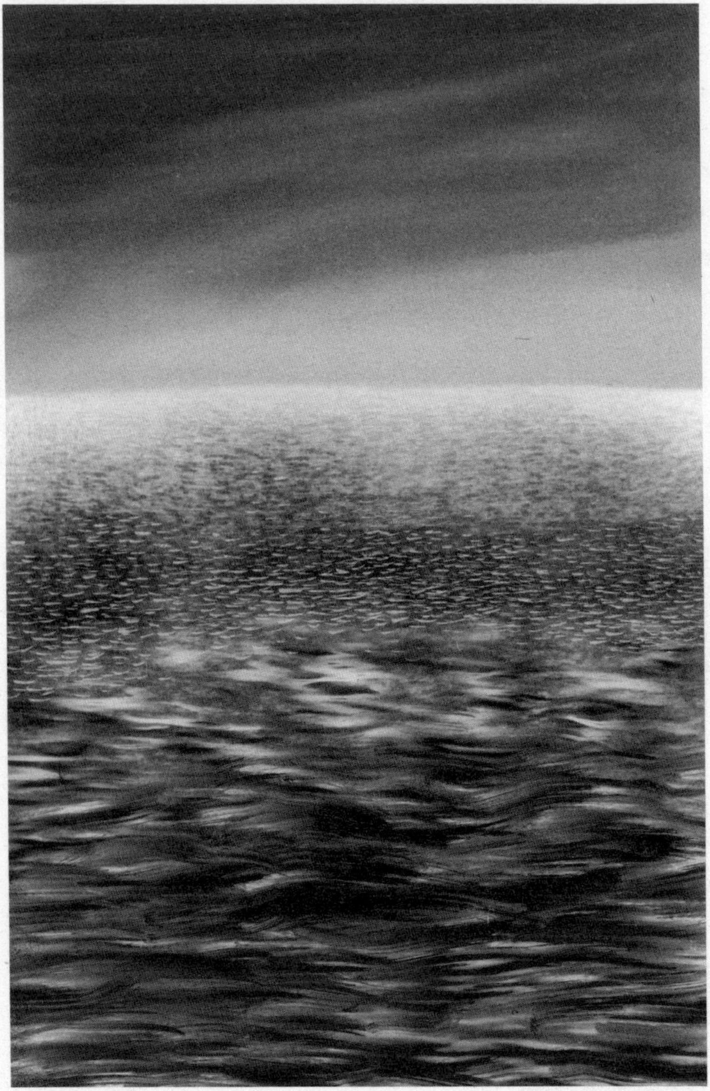

Suicide pervades, to the core, the clinical practice of psychiatry. The fear and the anxiety that attend every assessment made of risk, and the anger and the consternation that ensue following a self-inflicted death, cast a long shadow. Suicide and its aftermath are devastating to all involved, and to the responsible clinicians it represents a sense of profound failure. It haunts one for years, it undermines confidence, it carries with it a burden of self-reproach and helplessness. What could I have done to prevent this from happening? We should have known. We should have picked up the signals. Now it is too late.

I have known colleagues who have stopped practising in the aftermath of suicide. The blame, however ill-founded it might be, the emotional turmoil and the anxiety that this might happen yet again, weighs too heavily.

My first night on call as a trainee psychiatrist compelled me to face these daunting and painful issues. Night calls have always been difficult for me and I am sure for many of my colleagues. You are not able to withdraw, if only for a few hours, to reflect or to escape or to regain yourself. You are also alone. You are responsible. Anything can happen, and certainly in the early stages of training you have little reason to be confident that you will be able to cope with whatever crisis develops.

I had found the first few days at the beginning of my rotation predictably difficult. I was new to the hospital, there were unfamiliar routines and there were many members of staff with whom I needed to acquaint myself. There was also inevitably a degree of uncertainty about whether this was the right choice. I was embarking on a four-year training course in a speciality about which of course I could not know very much. This was in the UK and I was also needing to accustom myself to the often subtly different ways of thinking and doing things.

The first night call was on the fourth or fifth day of this project and I was anxious. I think there might also have been some degree of resentment that I was not to be granted the respite of the short time I felt I needed just to cope with the demands of my new job. The first few hours were relatively quiet and I had just finished a routine ward round when I received a call from the head nurse.

'You have to come to the admission ward, now!' he said, and there was a strain of urgency in this that intensified my feelings of apprehension.

'What is it?' I asked.

'Just come,' and again, 'now!'

I arrived in the ward to find a cluster of nurses staring at the closed door of a lavatory. Nobody said anything. It was not immediately clear to me what I was supposed to do. It also seemed curious why a doctor was required to open the door, or why a closed door should constitute an emergency. Yet clearly the nurses gazing at the door were fearful. The silence was ominous. The head nurse, who had previously appeared to me as a man of great confidence and ability, was now unsure of himself. It was disconcerting. He was fretful and indecisive. His staff turned to him. He turned to me. 'Doctor, you do it. Please,' he almost whispered, and it seemed to me for a moment absurdly as if he was asking me to do the honours. The group of observers stood back and I opened the door, knowing by then what was to confront us.

There is an appalling and confounding absence that surrounds a hanging body. We gazed upon our patient in horror. It is a vast stillness and a silence that extends beyond the lifeless body but binds us to it and shuts out the world. He was beyond us. He was dead, but in the confusion of emotions that engulfed us all it was difficult not to imagine in that inert form a reproach, a now silenced howl of rage against a world that had forsaken him. He had gone, but I think for many of us he was shouting at us: 'Why did you not help me?'

I had admitted him hours earlier. He was a middle-aged man who had been living alone on a farm some miles from the hospital. His brother had become concerned about his well-being. There was no history of mental illness but the brother had thought he had become depressed following the end of his marriage in divorce some months earlier. The brother had suggested to him that he should seek help and he had agreed with some reluctance to attend the outpatient clinic. I had seen him on the afternoon of his admission.

His manner was cautious but he was pleasant in a rather detached way towards me. I felt some sympathy from him, possibly owing to his seeing me as an inexperienced young doctor who could not possibly understand the darkness of the world that had come to envelop him.

His answers to my questions were vague and he gave an impression of being almost uninterested. He 'might' be depressed, he thought. It was a possibility, but 'to be expected' in the circumstances. With regard to the possibility of suicide he was evasive. He shrugged his shoulders and after a moment shook his head, but this was without conviction. There was a weariness about him. He was scarcely attending to me. He was preoccupied and remote.

Living alone and with little support, being middle-aged and being depressed did put him at risk of suicide. When I tentatively suggested an admission he did not refuse; nor did he appear to welcome this proposal. He did not seem to care. I explained the procedures to him and he signed the forms. I informed the nursing staff that the decision had been made to admit him out of concern that he posed a risk of suicide but I did not give an instruction that he should be under constant observation on a one-to-one basis. I did not think he posed that degree of risk. I was ignorant of the furious intent that suicide can demonstrate. I did not see him alive again and it was not possible for me not to think that I was responsible, and that by issuing more specific instructions I could have prevented his death.

There follows the dreaded responsibility of the telephone call to inform the family. Nobody had told me how I should do this, but it seems improbable anyway that there might be a right way, and that it is not always going to be awful. I have undertaken this miserable task on a number of occasions and it follows a curiously similar sequence: first the confusion, then the anger, then the grief.

'No … no … there has to be a mistake … it is not true … please tell me this is not true … this is not happening … no! … but … but he was in hospital … you admitted him because you were worried that he might do something … he was supposed to be safe in hospital … it can't be true … why did you allow this to happen … what sort of care is this … I don't believe this … tell me it is not true … I can't believe this … you tell me he is gone … that he is dead … that he hanged himself … no! … please … please tell me there has been some sort of mistake … please not my brother, not my son, not my father … not somebody who meant the whole world to me … this person I cannot imagine living without … and now you have let him die … how could you? … how could you let this happen?'

Then there is the legal process, the court hearings, the apportioning of blame, the protracted bureaucratic process that inevitably ensues and that might be imagined to attenuate the anger and grief but does not.

What did I do wrong? What did I miss? What could I have done to stop it? are constant and quite possibly inevitable refrains that attend the aftermath of a suicide.

This becomes more acute or painful the closer it is to you. A colleague at work started to drift away from us. There was nothing dramatic, no apparent crisis. He just seemed to lose interest in the work he was doing and an enthusiasm in his professional behaviour to which we had become accustomed. There were a few minor mistakes or perhaps oversights or lapses of judgement, but nothing that gave rise to a serious cause for concern. We suggested that he take some time off work. Perhaps there was a lot going on that we were unaware of and he should give himself time to sort things out.

He did not come to the clinic the next week and we chose to believe that he had heeded our advice and taken a few days off. His wife contacted our principal. He had been found in a remote area, some distance from his home. He was alive. Some children had found him in his car with a pipe leading from the exhaust to the interior. They had detached the pipe and opened the windows and he had revived. He returned home. He returned to work. What had happened was impossible. It was inconceivable that this husband and father and successful and highly respected professional person should seek to kill himself. His desperate act was denied.

He disappeared the next week. Again he was found, this time in a different place, but again close to death with a pipe leading from the exhaust into the vehicle. It then became difficult or irresponsible to ignore the fact that there was a grave crisis, but for reasons that were unfathomable to me he was admitted to a surgical ward in a private hospital. I can only think that it was considered unacceptable that a colleague should be admitted to the acute unit of the public hospital where I worked as a consultant. I don't know whether it was thought of as somehow shameful. I don't know whether the situation was deemed not sufficiently grave to consider such a radical intervention. I was not consulted or involved in any way in these decisions.

So with all the respect owing to a colleague and specialist physician he was admitted to a private suite in a surgical ward with no restriction on his movement. He promptly went to a local pharmacy where he procured a wide range of sedatives and opiates that he prescribed for himself. He consumed the lot, climbed to the top of the building in which the clinic was situated and threw himself to his death from the roof.

A turmoil of rage and grief and recriminations followed. How could this have been allowed to happen? All the signs had been there. What sort of nonsensical or wishful thinking was it that a doctor should be considered immune to desperation and to the risk of suicide? Why had his colleagues not seen what was going on – including a psychiatrist, for God's sake? Why had we not done anything? Even in anguished retrospect I have no idea what drove my colleague to his suicide. It seems clear that he was determined, and it is not at all clear whether more decisive and restrictive measures would have saved him.

This fierce resolve is mysterious and can be deceptive. Perhaps it is within us all to refuse to believe that somebody, whether it is a patient or a friend or a family member, has made a decision to end their lives. It appals us. It is unthinkable.

It is a curious and anomalous observation that in suicidal behaviour the most determined acts are not infrequently without apparent cause. Liam was a successful accountant, married, with a nine-year-old daughter. He set off for work one morning without, it seemed, a care in the world. The office phoned his wife towards midday saying that he had not arrived at work. It was most uncharacteristic of him not to inform the office if for whatever reason he would not be coming in. His wife went down to the garage of their home where she found her husband unconscious. He was lying in a pool of blood and in his hand was a knife with which he had slit his throat.

When I encountered him in the surgical ward he had fully regained consciousness, but spoke with difficulty because of the pressure bandages around his neck. He was babbling. He seemed excited to be alive. At that time, and on the many occasions afterwards when I spoke to both him and his wife, he could provide no explanation for his actions. He said there were no problems in his life. He was happily married. He loved his daughter dearly. He enjoyed his work. He was utterly mystified as to why, in such a violent manner, he had attempted to end his seemingly most fortunate life.

Peter was employed by the university in an administrative capacity. He too was happily married with a young family, and he too denied that there were any major problems in his life. The first time I met him he appeared to me as a character in a horror film. He was encased in plasters and splints. Pressure bandages enveloped his neck and forearms and his skull was protected by a helmet. He had first cut his throat. That was unsuccessful, so he had been admitted to a private clinic. There he had managed to dive head-first from the first floor into an atrium, fracturing his skull and his pelvis. After some days he had been allowed to leave the clinic for a few hours in the company of his wife. While her attention had been momentarily diverted he had used a screwdriver to pierce the fibrous compartments of both forearms and sever his radial arteries. When he finally got to us, now as an involuntary admission, he was elated. He seemed delighted to be alive. He was fascinated by the curious behaviour of the other patients on the ward. He wanted to engage with them and do whatever he could to help them, but they shrank away from him in horror at his bizarre appearance.

He could not explain his behaviour. I do not doubt that he tried to make sense of what he had done to himself. He had come desperately close to killing himself, but for years afterwards when I saw him in the outpatient clinic he remained bewildered by his actions. At no point did he ever seem depressed. He went back to work and to his family. When I last saw him before he returned to private care he was cheerful and seemed confident that there would be no recurrence of these unfathomable and violent events.

If any light or hope can be found in this profoundly sad expression of the human predicament, it might be in the way that, as these determined and desperate acts of self-harm arise in some, they as mysteriously pass. I remain nevertheless haunted by the events I have described.

39

HIV and madness

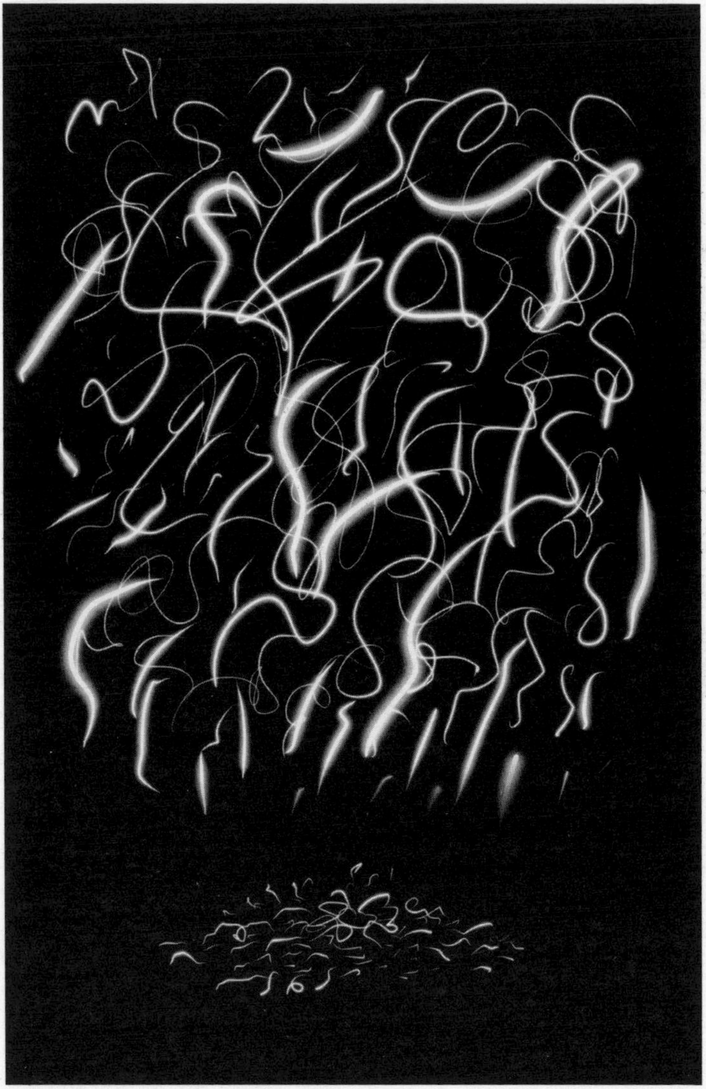

Mzamo is adrift. He is vacant. He is elsewhere but I have no idea where that is. Dishevelled, he gazes at us with a disconcerting impassivity from his chair. He does not appear to be in distress. He is emaciated. He is not agitated. Anger about being where he is does not appear to account for his disengagement with his surroundings. He answers our questions, but with a delay, and slowly, without emotion. He is apathetic.

'Mzamo, how are you coping? What's going on? How can we help you?' A long silence ensues. Can he hear us? Has he forgotten our questions? Is he beyond caring?

Then, quietly, with a degree of perplexity, almost to himself, he says, 'No, I am … all right … no problems … yes … it's all right.' And after a long pause, 'Thank you.'

There are a number of possibilities for us to consider and, as we so often preach to the students, it is unlikely that there is only one explanation. It is far more probable that there are a range of interacting factors that contribute to this rather enigmatic presentation.

Mzamo has Aids. He has a low CD4 count. He also has tuberculosis. He also has schizophrenia. He also, possibly to cope with these problems, has a long history of alcohol abuse.

He has lived with HIV for over fifteen years. How he contracted the illness is again open to a range of possible factors. At that time, there was much controversy about what might cause the illness, how it should be treated and, curiously, even whether it existed at all. Garlic and the African potato were proposed as remedies by the Ministry of Health. In this context it is quite possible that Mzamo either ignored his symptoms or delayed treatment.

The diagnosis of schizophrenia preceded the HIV. The self-neglect and the loss of any sense of self or control over his circumstances would certainly have rendered him vulnerable to infection. This would also have undermined his engagement with any treatment programme. Without support, it would perhaps have been expecting too much of him to adhere to the relatively complex treatment regimes of both schizophrenia and HIV. It therefore became grimly predictable that the HIV would develop into Aids and that, as a consequence of his impaired immunity, he would become afflicted with tuberculosis. Living alone, with little or no support from family or friends, it had then become even more improbable, or impossible, that he could have been expected to cope with living with HIV/Aids, schizophrenia and tuberculosis. It is not clear when alcohol became a problem, and that in itself is yet again a consequence of many likely factors.

He had moved many years previously from the Eastern Cape to the city in search of work. He had lost contact with his family and his community. The suspicions and social awkwardness of schizophrenia would have undermined the resources he had to seek support in a new and alien world. He had been unable to find regular work and was living in poverty in one of the many informal settlements that were developing on the peripheries of the city. In these dire circumstances it is unsurprising that he should seek solace in alcohol. In the shebeens there was at least some semblance of a community and the illusory hope of putting aside, at least for a while, the hopelessness of his predicament. It is again quite understandable that in these circumstances he should seek comfort in sex – and that given his isolation and his social unease this should have to be paid for. He had earned a small income from occasional, informal and unskilled work, and these pitiful amounts were spent on alcohol and prostitutes.

He had made some desultory attempts to attend the local clinics for his medication but this was for the HIV, not the schizophrenia. Even in his abject state he was fearful of being seen in the queue to receive psychiatric attention. The stigma of mental illness was greater than that of HIV/Aids. Predictably he relapsed.

He had been brought to the emergency unit by the police who had found him wandering in the traffic in the city centre. It did not seem to them that he was attempting to kill himself. He seemed confused and he was unable to give a clear account of himself. He was examined and the diagnoses of HIV/Aids and pulmonary tuberculosis were confirmed. Treatment was restarted. Probably not knowing what to do with him the medical staff referred him onward to our service.

This is often a source of rancour. The registrars perform a more or less ritual exchange. The psychiatrists will accuse the emergency physicians of dumping the patient. The medical team will say they are overwhelmed, they have done what they can, and they do not have the resources to assess and manage psychiatric disorders. The social workers usually join in the fray. This is time-consuming and enervating, and if a stalemate develops the consultant becomes involved. At this stage there does not seem to be an option. Time is being wasted and goodwill is being undermined. I accept the transfer. Mzamo eventually finds himself in our ward, baffled, disoriented, stupefied by the sedative medications he has been given in the emergency unit.

Perhaps the most striking feature is his slowness. For this there are many possible explanations. The most obvious is the sedative medication, given regularly in emergency units for fear of the havoc that can be caused by a psychotic patient disrupting the emergency care of ill patients. In this circumstance sedation does not seem likely. He is not drowsy. He is alert, but is not with us. Delirium is always a source of great anxiety. It can be life-threatening and for Mzamo there are many possible causes, including the HIV or the tuberculosis or both involving his brain, or any other infective agent due to his compromised immune system. The slowness could be explained by depression. There are many reasons for him to be depressed. People often do not say they are depressed. This tends to occur in the more severe forms of depression. If you are very depressed and consider your situation to be hopeless, what is the point of telling anybody that you are depressed? It seems very possible to us that this is what Mzamo might be thinking and feeling. This sense of futility could in all likelihood be confounded by his being in a very unfamiliar environment, surrounded by inquisitive strangers speaking a language of which he has only the slightest grasp, asking inane questions like 'How are you?' and 'What is the matter?' – as if he knew or could even begin to make sense of what has happened to him.

The slowness could be accounted for by the schizophrenia or by the medications that have been used to treat it. Delusions of persecution can induce a wariness that might be expressed in caution and slowness. The slowness might be due to distraction owing to auditory hallucinations or intrusive commenting voices. Catatonia is a severe form of schizophrenia that can present with a dramatic slowness to the point of immobility and mutism. The negative forms of schizophrenia – the social withdrawal and emotional flatness and loss of volition often associated with cognitive problems, including impaired attention – are further possibilities that we need to consider. Antipsychotic medications can cause slowness in different ways, probably most commonly through sedation or by the curious Parkinsonian side-effects induced by many of these agents, particularly when used in high doses.

Another possibility to account for Mzamo's rather inscrutable presentation of being there and yet not being there is some form of dementia. We do not know his age but he is probably in his forties, which would be early for the more common forms of dementia. Excessive consumption of alcohol is a not-uncommon cause of dementia at this age. This is associated with a general lack of self-care, including inadequate nutrition – and, as happens so often in states of drunkenness, violence and repeated head injuries, all of which could be contributing to Mzamo's slowness and possible dementia.

The most probable explanation is HIV/Aids. This has become one of the more common causes of dementia in younger people. A characteristic feature of this kind of dementia is slowness due to the damage caused by the virus to particular parts of the brain. Mzamo's apathy could be explained by any one of these factors. It is more probable that some or all of these possible causative factors are interacting to produce what seems to be an intractable problem and a deeply sad and lonely predicament.

HIV can affect the brain in a number of ways. It can cause an encephalopathy or inflammation of the central nervous system that would usually present as a delirium, an altered state of consciousness. Through a suppression of the immune system the virus may cause a wide range of secondary viral, fungal, parasitic and bacterial infections of the brain, including tuberculosis. It may cause a number of malignancies or rare cancers of the brain. It may cause dementias. Antiretroviral treatments may cause many psychological and neuropsychiatric problems. The associations of HIV and madness are complex and profuse.

There is another non-biological and more figurative way in which madness pertains to HIV. In the early part of this century President Thabo Mbeki declares that the human immunodeficiency virus does not cause Aids. This is in defiant opposition to the scientific and medical consensus of the time. He is supported in this bizarre claim by the Minister of Health, Dr Manto Tshabalala-Msimang. 'Western medicine' is rejected. Aids activism represents a neocolonialist intervention, Mbeki declares. Tshabalala-Msimang commends as a cure *ubhejane*, garlic, lemon and beetroot. She becomes known as Dr Beetroot. As a result of the denialism of these two politicians it is estimated in a report by Harvard University's School of Public Health that approximately 350 000 South Africans succumb to preventable deaths.

My closest friend during my school and undergraduate years died of Aids. He was not in denial of his status. He had perhaps been in a quite mad denial of the consequences of the grave risks he took and in the apparent belief of his invulnerability. He excelled at everything he undertook. At school he was top of the class in most subjects. He captained the first teams in cricket and rugby and athletics. He occupied leadership positions and was held in high esteem by teachers and scholars. He continued to flourish at university. He was a star. He soared, it seemed, above us and beyond us.

His secret behaviour confounded me. He was a medical student. He knew all about HIV and Aids. He knew the risks he was taking with apparent abandon. He seemed compelled to test the limits, to fly as close as he could to the sun. I was unable to stop him. He laughed. Everything was a big adventure. His sexual exploits appeared to be all the more thrilling to him because he knew of the dangers. I think he was perhaps scornful of my concern and my caution. I found it increasingly difficult to be with him. What had at one time seemed almost heroically daring and creative now seemed wilfully destructive. We drifted apart. He flew on, further and further, more and more dangerously, until it became inevitable that he would burn and crash. When I last saw him shortly before his death he was weak and angry. Anger also confused my grief. It was such a terrible waste. He had been my best friend and I will never know what dark and mysterious forces led him to his early death.

There is nevertheless something in this story that is perhaps understandable and that is not confined to my friend's trajectory. In the sexual act we abandon ourselves. We seek to lose ourselves. We are heedless of the consequences. Sex is dangerous. It requires taking risks. In our relinquishing all control in a brief state of rapture it is a moment of madness. It is outside reason and care and caution. The cruelty and sadness of it is that, in that moment of bliss and transcendence, there should fall the shadow of possible disease and destruction. In the Garden of Eden there will always be a snake, hissing and whispering in the leaves of the apple tree, driving us mad by burdening us with the preposterous notion that we might not be entirely in control of our lives, that innocence is transitory, and paradise ephemeral.

Mzamo is now beyond this madness. He is beyond caring and beyond seeking. He can be helped, to some extent. The tuberculosis can be treated. The schizophrenia can be managed and the HIV can be contained. He will be transferred to a home where his complex regime of medications can be supervised. He will receive a disability grant. It is unknowable whether, in the oblivion of his dementia, he might find some form of sanctuary.

40

Huntington's disease, syphilis and other tragedies of the damaged brain

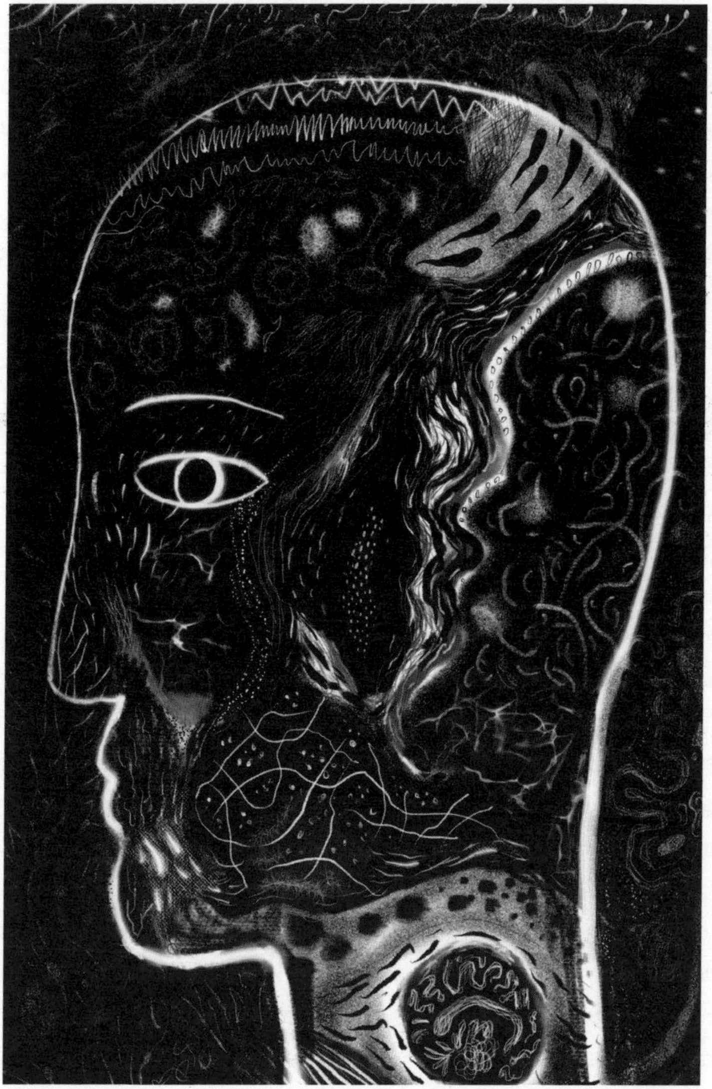

He is writhing about in a cot bed. He does not register us in any way. He makes curious distressing keening sounds. He beats his head against the side of the cot. He is wearing incontinence pads. His movements are purposeless. His eyes are vacant. He is my age. We were at school together. He was a champion tennis player.

The first indication had been a slight clumsiness. Nobody thought much of it at the time. He was in his early forties. Perhaps this was to be expected as we grow older. Perhaps it would pass. Then there were small, transitory lapses of attention. Perhaps this was due to stresses at work. Others mentioned similar problems. It was thought to be innocuous. It did not seem sinister. His wife described the movement and coordination problems becoming more marked and persistent. He became self-conscious about this. It seemed as if he might be drunk. His children, then in early adolescence, grew anxious and embarrassed. He had always paid scrupulous attention to his health. He had continued with the tennis and played competitively but now, to his great dismay, he was unable to perform what had been for him the most basic manoeuvres.

Alarm mounted. He appeared to have difficulty finding the appropriate words and his speech was sometimes slurred. At work his colleagues expressed a concern that some of the decisions he made were ill-judged. This was affecting his performance and the business was beginning to suffer. They encouraged him to take leave. Initially he refused. He seemed to lack insight into the increasing gravity of the situation. Eventually there was no alternative. His colleagues insisted. As the movement and the cognitive problems persisted and seemed to worsen it became apparent – to the great distress of his family – that it was increasingly unlikely that he would be able to return to work. Financial anxieties now compounded their fears. Then his father, a man in his late seventies, began to show the same symptoms. It eventually became clear that both were afflicted with Huntington's disease. I think this must be one of the most cruel of all neurological disorders, and the reason for this is its genetics.

The tragedy that was engulfing this family was in some ways unusual for Huntington's. It is an inherited disorder. The transmission is autosomally dominant, indicating that the children of an affected person, regardless of gender, have a one-in-two chance of inheriting the illness. With regard to my school friend and now my patient, the diagnosis was perhaps delayed because there was no apparent family history of Huntington's. It is recognised that symptoms may appear at earlier ages in succeeding generations, and it also seems probable that, with increasing longevity, a family history might become evident in an aging parent who would have otherwise died of another natural cause.

The son and daughter stand with their mother and me at the end of their father's bed, observing in dismay his agitated figure, having to confront his inaccessibility and their own threatened futures. Both are about to finish their schooling and both have plans to go to university. There has been no reason to doubt their bright and happy and successful trajectories, which is in the nature of their age, and now this has all been thrown into turmoil. They know they have a one-in-two chance of inheriting this illness and becoming like the demented father upon whom they now gaze in pity and horror. They are having to contemplate not only the loss of their father but possibly of their own futures. The mother holds the hands of both her children. She is a source of immense strength and support for them. I am filled with a sense of wonder by the extraordinary resilience and the grace shown by this mother and grieving wife and by many others who cope in some inspiring way with what seems to be a dreadful and unendurable situation.

It is possible to test whether one is carrying the Huntington's gene, but this raises a wide range of difficult issues that are all the more complicated and agonising for a young person. A positive test confers an inevitability. There will no longer be a tentative optimism allowed by a degree of uncertainty. My experience has been that for the most part the test is refused, and this is understandable. Why should a young person choose to close down hope, to live thereafter in a constant state of apprehension that any twitch or tremor might herald the onset of the disease and an inevitable decline towards dementia and death? When a decision is made to be tested, it is usually in the context of a young woman wanting to know whether she should start a family and being determined not to pass the gene on to her children. It is a grave burden to bear.

The family of a colleague was affected by this wretched illness. An elder brother had died in a car accident, and it was suspected that he had begun to detect the early signs of the illness in himself and had chosen to end his life. My colleague's whole life had been lived in the shadow of Huntington's. His ambition was to study medicine and specialise in neurology with the aim of finding a cure for the illness that had destroyed so many members of his family. For this reason he agreed to the test, arguing understandably that it would be futile to embark on such a long and arduous course if the symptoms of the illness were to make it impossible for him to realise his wishes. It was a very courageous thing to have done. The test was negative. He became a doctor. He has not discovered a cure for Huntington's. At present, it is not foreseeable.

Kobus is in good spirits. He greets the students cheerfully. He seems to enjoy the company of young people and he responds to their enquiries enthusiastically. I have asked the group to spend some time with him before the ward round. We reconvene five minutes later. I ask him whether he has met them before. He appears to think this is a ridiculous question. He is nevertheless polite and says, as if not wanting to offend, 'No, I don't think so. No, I have never met these young people.' They have spent about ten minutes with him. They are startled. In their earlier conversation with him, there is nothing at all to suggest that he has no short-term memory. He is amicable. He is engaging. He seems to be well. Compared to the other patients on the ward they have seen, he appears to be intact. There does not seem to be anything the matter. The only slight problem is his vagueness about the reasons for his admission, and this they probably register only in retrospect.

This encapsulated phenomenon of short-term memory loss is fascinating and disquieting. All other cognitive faculties remain intact. Kobus has retained all his social skills. He speaks fluently and articulately. There appears to be no damage and yet he is incapacitated. He is hospital-bound.

When asked how he spent the weekend Kobus for a moment seems baffled. We know he has spent the weekend as he has spent every weekend on the ward. He has alienated himself from his family and his friends. There is nobody willing to take him out of the hospital. The moment passes and Kobus then embarks on a lengthy and delighted account of his exciting weekend: he had been on a hunting trip with friends. He animatedly describes the fire they made in the evening, the meat they cooked, the stories they told, and yes, the large amount of beer and spirits they consumed.

Confronted fleetingly with a quite possibly terrifying sense of nothingness, Kobus retrieves long-term memories. He moves through life in the continuous moment of the present. His not knowing what he was thinking or doing moments previously renders him unable to function. He has no story. The whole rambling edifice of a personal narrative collapses into the vacancy of the immediate moment. He can make no sense of where he is and why he is here and what is going on around him because there is no past and there is no future. He cannot move from point A to point B. He is trapped forever in the confined world of point A, the non-contingent present.

He may be helpless, but he uses the other parts of his battered intelligence to hide this in confabulations. There is only a moment when his bewilderment shows – just before he is able to fabricate a world that makes some sense to him.

It is a mystery why alcohol should ruin the very small and specific parts of the brain, the mammillary bodies, that form part of the diencephalon adjacent to the midbrain. With continued alcohol use the damage spreads. Alcohol is one of the more common causes of dementia before the age of sixty-five. Kobus is not demented. The damage and the deficit are localised. Had he continued his excesses, he would in all likelihood have become demented, but he forgot who he was, he forgot the alcohol and he forgot what he had done to himself.

Dirk had also been profoundly affected by damage to a very specific part of his brain. I saw him regularly in one of the local community clinics. He had no problems with memory. He always greeted me pleasantly and by name. A familiar routine ensued. He was quite well, thank you. He was living with a girlfriend and she was also doing well, thank you. He was calm and composed and then quite suddenly he would burst into tears. The tears were profuse and appeared to be beyond his control. This embarrassed him greatly. In between the sobbing, scarcely audibly, he would say, 'I am sorry, Doctor. I am so sorry. I can't control it. I am not depressed. There is nothing wrong with me. It's just this crying. I can't stop it. It just comes over me suddenly. I can't stop it. My girlfriend gets angry with me. She doesn't believe me. She says there must be something wrong but there isn't.' Then, quite suddenly, the tears abate. He composes himself and smiles at me. 'I am fine, really. It's just this crying that I can't seem to control. It is completely unpredictable and it's embarrassing and annoying. People don't understand that it is because of the accident. They think there is something wrong with me. People don't cry for no reason.'

Many years earlier Dirk had been involved in a motorbike accident. He had suffered a head injury and fractured his pelvis. After some months, he appeared to have recovered completely from these injuries, except for this one problem: an emotional incontinence that baffled and exasperated him. As a consequence of the closed head injury damage had been done to the inferior aspects of the frontal cortex. This highly evolved part of the brain mediates inhibition. His uncontrollable weeping was the expression of a disinhibition arising from the disruption of neurological circuits in this localised part of the brain.

There is no other overt indication of damage; curiously this causes much distress to those who are affected. There is no sign of a head injury. There is no paralysis nor any other dramatic feature to account for their changed behaviour. They have just lost control, or that is what people are thinking, and that is shameful. There is one neurological signal of injury to this part of the brain and that is a loss of olfaction, the capacity to smell, due to damage to the olfactory nerve fibres that pass through the base of the skull into the nasal cavity. It is not overt, but it is useful as an objective indication of damage to the brain. In a persisting dualistic way of thinking, it is curious that patients may be reassured by being informed that their changed behaviour can be attributed to brain damage rather than psychological causes.

Disinhibition following a head injury has other repercussions that can cause further harm. Alcohol may be consumed to excess, leading to aggression and violence and an increased risk of another head injury being sustained. Sexual disinhibition may lead to unwanted pregnancies or sexually transmitted infections. In this respect, HIV/Aids is a particular cause for concern as the impulsivity resulting from a head injury would make the necessarily scrupulous adherence to treatment improbable. Sexual disinhibition may also be manifested in many dementias. There is no insight into the gaucheness and the gross inappropriateness of this behaviour. The suffering is borne by others. This is very often the daughter who has to witness the ghastly attempts of her aged demented mother to flirt with a bewildered young doctor in the poignant and deluded belief that she has returned to her sexually alluring, younger self.

More diffuse injuries have more devastating effects, and this applies particularly to traumatic head injuries. The devastation is because these injuries are common and too often affect young people, ruining their and their families' lives. It is every parent's nightmare to receive a call in the middle of the night to inform them of the accident. John or Sophie or Xolisi has been out celebrating his or her birthday with friends or their graduation or matric results and maybe somebody has been irresponsible and had a few drinks before driving or maybe it was somebody else's fault but in seconds everything falls appallingly apart. There will be no university, no family, no happiness, no future, no sadness even, except for others' – just an enduring emptiness and loss. Traumatic brain injuries are among the more common causes of dementia in young people.

Syphilis is difficult because the early signs can resolve spontaneously, without treatment, only to reappear in some unfortunate person years later, wreaking havoc in the brain.

I saw Jack for a few years in the outpatient clinic of the hospital before referring him to the local community clinic when it became clear that there was not much more I could do for him. He had been treated for the neurosyphilis that had ruined him. He was demented, but the progression had been halted. He was calm and appeared to be contented. He was vacant. There was no problem. He had no complaints. There was nothing wrong with him. He did not know why his family was making all this fuss. He was quite capable of looking after himself.

He was not, and it was to my great relief and that of the family that he agreed without complaint to being moved to a supervised home. The blandness, his passive acquiescence and apparent unconcern, were part of the dementia but in this respect were to his advantage. He adapted in his way. He appears to be at peace in the world. He is not agitated. He is not in distress. He drifts on.

I have no idea what he is thinking, but it is just possible that in some way his dementia is protecting him from the pain of having lost his mind.

41

Meaning and madness

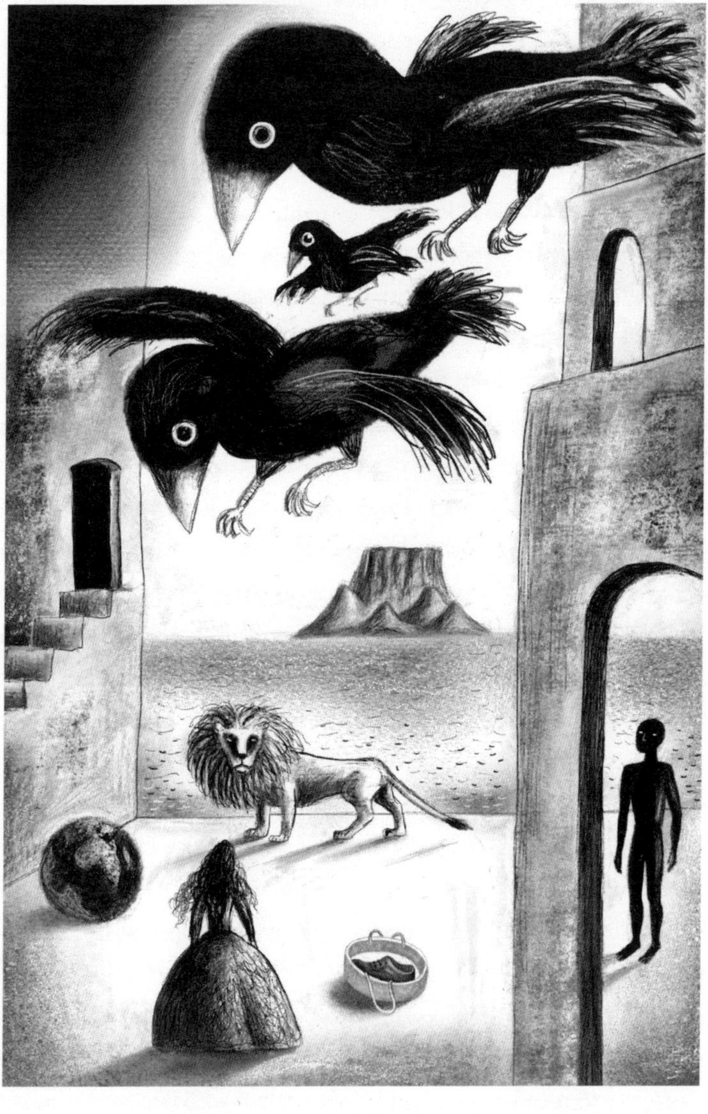

At the Monday-morning feedback meeting I am informed by the nursing staff that there are three Mandelas on the ward. They are behaving in a courteous, dignified way towards one another. There is no dispute as to who the true Mandela might be. They appear to respect the choice that each has made to be an eminent and revered figure. There has never been a Jacob Zuma on our ward. The ex-president is currently facing charges of corruption. He is not a popular figure in our refracted world. Some time ago, a very large and fierce black man from the Democratic Republic of the Congo was admitted to the high care unit insisting he was Helen Zille, the premier of the province at the time. This was curious because Helen Zille is a middle-aged white woman. It is also surprising that a recent immigrant from central Africa should have known who the premier is, and that he should have chosen to be her.

Choice is not generally a consideration in psychoses. You don't choose to be psychotic. Things happen to you over which you have no control. These things are usually bad, and it is unimaginable that such adverse experiences should be willingly sought. I do not think a psychosis is chosen, but I do think it is possible that, at some level, there is a degree of agency regarding the content of delusions. The choice to be a Mandela, for example, rather than a Zuma I believe is not random. It is not without meaning. These are two political figures who symbolise very different philosophies and moralities. The one features on our ward and the other does not. At any one time, an array of doctors, teachers, healers and others might be considered to have in common a wish to make the world a better place. I think our patients want the world to be safer and kinder and, in their strange and deluded ways, they believe that by being who they are they can possibly help themselves. Being a doctor, however mad, puts you in a position to help others and yourself, and that in itself brings hope.

I struggle to recall any patient in our system who believed he was evil, or was in any way at ease with this perception of himself. A young man was admitted to the high care unit because he was considered to be at high risk of harming himself. He had come to believe that he had killed his family. This caused him great anguish and he insisted that the only way this calamity could end would be for him to be killed in turn. However deeply mired our patients were in their private psychotic worlds, for the most part a discernible theme was evident in their aspiring to help themselves and others, and perhaps to do good. This man believed that he had done something that was terribly wrong and he wanted justice, even though that might require his own death.

Thabo was brought to the hospital by the police. He had presented himself at the Houses of Parliament earlier in the day and declared to the bemused security officers that he had come to take over the government that in his mind was corrupt and incompetent. It is not clear why this should lead to the conclusion that he was mentally ill but he was referred to our unit to be assessed. He was not an angry man. He was not violent in any way. For him overthrowing the government was more of a duty than a self-righteous insurrection. We did not think he was dangerous and he was moved to an open ward. I found him sitting at the fence looking at the birds on the river. He said, 'Our time will come. We have to be patient. My army of birds are awaiting my command. Then we will take over the government. My birds are ready. Our time will come.' He was calm. He was at peace with himself. He had a plan and he believed it was a just plan. The birds drifted in the shallow waters of the river, unperturbed.

At a biological level the experience of psychosis might be imagined as noise. A complex array of interacting factors contribute to this final pathway of disintegration. These might include a number of genetic variants – none of which is sufficient in isolation to precipitate the illness – epigenetic factors and adverse events in early and late childhood. A common precipitating insult in our practice is the abuse of substances, usually cannabis or methamphetamines. These toxic processes appear to disrupt the very precise and complex interplay of neurotransmitters and receptors in the central nervous system, leading to a disorganisation of the synchrony of neuronal networks and the experience of madness or mere noise. The delicately embroidered, elegantly folded fabrics of the mind are torn apart.

In this state, all is noise and chaos and devoid of meaning. It is difficult to imagine: our lives are so much made up of light and sound and thoughts and feelings that form meaningful patterns and which help us to make sense of our lives and may grant us pleasure. The patient experiencing a psychotic episode is robbed of these harmonies. We cannot know the mind of another, and certainly not the mind of a psychotic other, but we can imagine that such noise, such a dissolution of meaning, would be intolerable. In this context it becomes understandable that a person in such a state should urgently seek to find or construct meanings and, in this process, to employ themes that are culturally or spiritually familiar – albeit often in deeply strange ways, given the disorder of mind.

The formation of a delusion might therefore represent the emergence of a struggle for restoration, an attempted reframing of a terrifying and meaningless event into something that might just begin to make sense and restore a degree of control. If this might be so, we need to think very carefully about the ways in which we intervene. The focus of attention would then shift from simply eliminating or suppressing the symptoms of psychosis to reducing the significance or the control these symptoms have over a person's life – and the person's associated distress.

One critical step in this process is to re-imagine the symptom not merely as a sign of a pathological process but as an endeavour to find meaning and regain control. This would entail acknowledging rather than dismissing these often bewildering symptoms. I have no idea why this man from the DRC should come to believe that he is the white female premier of the province. I have more of an understanding of why the others have become Mandela, but they do share an aspiration of being in power and holding authority. In this respect, these delusions can be imagined as strategies for coping with otherwise unbearable feelings of helplessness and hopelessness.

'I need the drones for my mining projects ... I will be opening up a number of silicon mines in Brazil ... it's no problem ... the land is there for the taking ... you just take out the silicon and you wash it ... it is no problem ...' In a country where ownership of land is a vexed and politically fraught issue, this is a pleasant – if facile – solution. On the other side of a vast ocean there is land that is simply there for the taking. It also contains great riches. It is a fleetingly sustaining fantasy that finds concrete but temporary form in a delusion that is harmless.

Marius and Joan are sitting on a bench in the shade of a pine tree, holding hands in a contented intimacy. They are gazing at the birds on the river. There is a curiously serene and dignified demeanour about them, a stillness that is unusual in psychotic states. She is the Queen of England and he is her rather bewildered Prince. She is the authority and she bears herself with regal grace. Marius is shambolic in appearance and does not seem to be inclined to make much effort in being royal. He just goes along with it, I think for Joan's benefit.

She does not bother too much with this lack of enthusiasm on his part. I think she is grateful for the companionship. They look after each other in their own way. They glide along in their gentle madness with dignity. They are allowed to be who they choose to be. Nobody says to them, 'You are not the queen. You are not a prince. You are just mad old people.' They are not mocked. They are treated with some deference. There seems to be a shared belief that nothing is to be gained by taking away their delusion of nobility. It would be cruel, and there would be nothing to put in its place.

Simon was admitted after assaulting his mother. He worked in an embassy and had come to believe that listening devices had been installed in his office. This belief gradually increased in intensity and shifted to his home. He became convinced that his movements in all the rooms of the house he shared with his mother were being observed, and then that not only his movements but his thoughts were being monitored by some sinister and unknown organisation. I think he was trying to explain to his mother that, owing to the nature of his psychotic illness, his precarious sense of his self as being private had broken down, and that this understandably angered and frightened him. His poor mother became agitated and intolerant. She had been through this too many times before. She told us she no longer had the patience to listen to his crazy ravings. She said she was exhausted by his recurrent breakdowns and no longer had the reserves to attempt to understand what he was going through.

She told him he was ill and that he needed to be in hospital. Her dismissal of what to him was a terrifying reality had maddened him. It was this refusal to acknowledge his ordeal, he said, rather than the invasion of his privacy that had tipped the balance. In a fury of exasperation he had hit her, and now he was ashamed of what he had done. If only she had been able to believe him, or at least hear him, this would not have happened, he believed. His mother said she could not understand what he was saying to her. She was no longer willing to try to understand. It was meaningless. It was just this terrible illness and why could he not accept it?

This loss of hope and meaning is also described by those in severe states of depression. Moletsi said to me – after he had recovered, because in the midst of his illness he had been mute – 'There was no colour, no light and shade. There was no value to anything. There was nothing to give me direction or purpose. There was no meaning to anything. That was perhaps the worst of it, the loss of meaning, and with it hope.'

Whether it is through God or the ancestors, or whether it arises from our own needs, there is, within us all – whether or not we suffer from some form of mental illness – a need to find meaning in our lives, however meaningless that might be in some other implacable order of things.

Epilogue

The need for hope

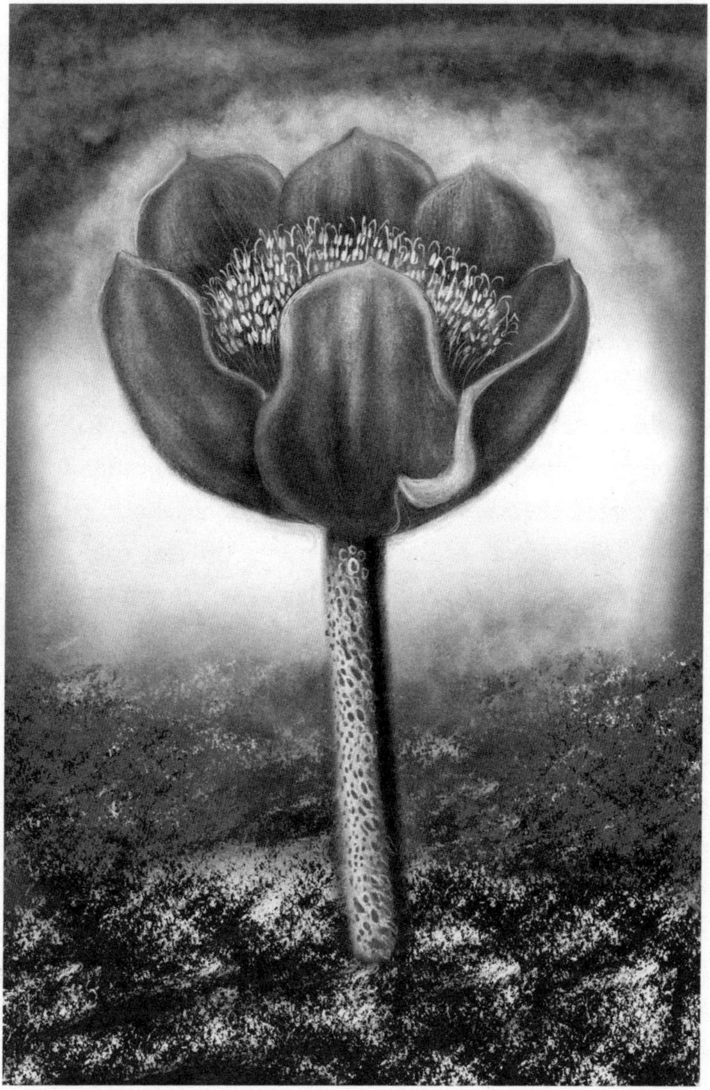

Hope is ephemeral. Hope is elusive. It is fragile. It is without reason. It is something to which we resort when there is no hope.

I am not sure how I would have coped in the hospital for as long as I did without hope.

On Monday morning, we gather in the nursing station to discuss the new admissions. There have been ten over the weekend. Sibusiso is back, having been discharged only six weeks ago. He was well when he left. Then, according to his mother, he stopped the medication after about two weeks and started to use methamphetamines. Despondency descends upon us. What are we doing? What are we hoping to achieve? It seems we are just patching things up. The nursing staff are demoralised. They say they are understaffed and the female members say they don't feel safe at night. All complain that they can't do their jobs properly because they have to fill in too many forms. The social worker is disgruntled. She says she has more important things to do than fill in application forms for disability grants. The occupational therapist says she cannot possibly provide an adequate service as she is on her own covering two wards. She says the nursing staff must help her but they say they cannot because they are occupied with their own duties. The occupational therapist says then the patients will become bored and frustrated and start fighting and it will just make things all the more difficult to manage. There is an awkward and sullen silence.

I receive a call from the bed manager. She is very considerate but there is a plea in her voice. 'Please,' she says, 'there are thirty-five patients now on the waiting list. I am under a lot of pressure. Is there anything you could possibly do?' She is politely asking me to discharge as many patients as soon as possible to create space for at least some of these thirty-five patients. They are being accommodated in the emergency units of hospitals and clinics in the greater urban area. If they need admission to our unit I know they are causing havoc. They will be harassing the nurses and disrupting emergency procedures and making everybody very angry with psychiatric patients.

'I will do what I can,' I say to the bed manager, having little idea how I am to discharge safely any of the severely disturbed young men currently in our wards.

The clinical psychologist weighs in with an angry contribution. She is disabled and the hospital management has not yet been able to organise the necessary assistance for her. She is extraordinarily determined and resilient but she says she does not think she will be able to attend these meetings for much longer. There is more silence. Gloom envelops us. I am the nominal leader of this group. I know I need to do something to stop this unhappy mood but what that might be is not apparent. Nobody told us at any stage of our training that maintaining morale would be an important part of our responsibilities.

A weary defeatism now looms in the confines of the nursing station. The patients peer anxiously through the partition, as if sensing our predicament. We are on the verge of being confounded by the futility of it all. I become a little bit desperate on occasions like this and absurdly bring cakes to the meetings, as if that could make things better.

I need to instil hope, if not in the expectation that things will get better then at least in that what we are doing, however inadequate, might just be helpful, to some degree, in some way. It is what we need to think, or believe, in order to cope and not become downcast.

Hope is a form of seeking. We seek food and sex and shelter to survive. We need hope to survive.

Frequently I don't know how families cope. I don't know how Sibusiso's mother manages after he has been admitted yet again, for the same predictable and exasperating reasons. He gets well, promising to take his medication. He promises to attend the local clinic. He promises not to use drugs. 'Don't worry,' he laughs, wanting to reassure us, 'I have learnt my lesson. You are not going to see me again in this hospital. Never again! I need to get on with my life.' He has said this again and again, and now his mother sits in our interview room, gazing balefully at us, angry and disconsolate.

'Why don't you doctors keep him? You know what is going to happen. You know he will come back. He is clever. He knows what to say so that you will release him.' We have been through this before. She knows that we have no option other than to discharge her son. Another oppressive silence ensues. She seems reluctant to leave. 'Tell me, Doctor, is this a life-long illness? Is this going to go on until I die and then what will happen to him? The people in the community say that there is no cure for this and that he will never get better. Is there any hope?'

'Yes, of course there is. We don't know what the future holds for Sibusiso. Anything is possible. There is always hope.'

Uncertainty is difficult to live with, but it does provide a space for hope, and certainty in this circumstance would be false. 'It is true that there is no cure but that goes for many illnesses, such as heart disease or diabetes, and people learn to live with these problems,' I say. But diabetes is not like schizophrenia. It does not change the way you are. It does not cause you to scream at imagined voices or turn violently against your mother in the belief that she has become a witch.

It is necessary and respectful to be honest, but honesty does not need to foreclose on hope. We need to find some creative balance between acceptance that is not resignation and hopefulness that is not hopeless. Our patients and their families guide us.

Sibusiso will leave with his mother. They will go back across the river. She will not give up hope. This is what happens in the great majority of such circumstances. There is a profound and inspiring dignity and strength in the resilience that these mothers show. It is mostly the mothers. Perhaps they will have to put some things aside. There will need to be a re-evaluation of priorities and a reconsideration of what is most important in life. It is probable that Sibusiso will not become the man she had once dreamed he might be, but she tells us that will not stop her loving him. He is her son and he will always be her son and she refuses to give up hope.

I don't think Sibusiso has the intention of deceiving us. I do not doubt that he wants to be well and get on with his life. I don't think he has given up hope. He cannot afford to. I hope he will find direction in his life and some meaning that will give him purpose, however strange and different that might be. Hope is not fragile or desperate. Hopefully it will provide him with the strength he will need, and we all need.

Beyond hopelessness and reason and madness there is only hope.

Acknowledgements

I want to thank the following people who have, in many different ways, contributed to the development of the ideas expressed in this book, for which, in the end, I must hold sole responsibility: Tony Morphet, Ingrid de Kok, Nigel Penn, Sean Kaliski, Sue Hawkridge, John Parker, Penny Busetto, Judy Gathercole, Berit Maxwell, Johan Liebenberg, Lara Foot, Steve Reid, Leslie Swartz and all my colleagues in the Department of Psychiatry and Mental Health in the Health Sciences Faculty of the University of Cape Town.

I wish to express my gratitude and admiration for the nursing staff and all other staff working at Valkenberg Hospital in Cape Town, who work with impressive care, dedication and skill in often very difficult circumstances.

I am thankful to Jeremy Boraine of Jonathan Ball Publishers for encouraging me to embark on this project, to Caren van Houwelingen for her supervision of the process, and to Angela Voges for her careful attention to the arduous process of editing the text, and for her engagement with the themes I have sought to articulate.

I will always be in gratitude to my family, Fiona, Anna and Clara, who have brought light and beauty into my life and who have continued to sustain and inspire me. I am in wonder at the illustrations for the text created by Fiona: they vividly and mysteriously express what reaches beyond words.

I wish to acknowledge with great respect my patients and their families with whom I have worked for so many, to me, fortunate years, and who have prompted me to write this book and to whom it is dedicated.

Sean Baumann

Sean Baumann worked for twenty-five years as a consultant to the male acute service at Valkenberg Hospital in Cape Town and was a senior lecturer in the Department of Psychiatry and Mental Health at UCT. He currently holds an honorary position in the department. He obtained degrees in the arts and in medicine and qualified as a specialist psychiatrist in London, UK. His interests are psychotic illnesses, specifically the schizophrenia spectrum disorders, and chronic pain. He is the editor of *Primary Care Psychiatry: A Practical Guide for Southern Africa* (1998, 2007, 2015). His cantata *Madness: Songs of Hope and Despair* was performed at the Baxter Theatre in Cape Town in 2017.